Mometrix
TEST PREPARATION

AF271545

CMC®
Secrets Study Guide

Introduction

Thank you for purchasing this resource! You have made the choice to prepare yourself for a test that could have a huge impact on your future, and this guide is designed to help you be fully ready for test day. Obviously, it's important to have a solid understanding of the test material, but you also need to be prepared for the unique environment and stressors of the test, so that you can perform to the best of your abilities.

For this purpose, the first section that appears in this guide is the **Secret Keys**. We've devoted countless hours to meticulously researching what works and what doesn't, and we've boiled down our findings to the five most impactful steps you can take to improve your performance on the test. We start at the beginning with study planning and move through the preparation process, all the way to the testing strategies that will help you get the most out of what you know when you're finally sitting in front of the test.

We recommend that you start preparing for your test as far in advance as possible. However, if you've bought this guide as a last-minute study resource and only have a few days before your test, we recommend that you skip over the first two Secret Keys since they address a long-term study plan.

If you struggle with **test anxiety**, we strongly encourage you to check out our recommendations for how you can overcome it. Test anxiety is a formidable foe, but it can be beaten, and we want to make sure you have the tools you need to defeat it.

1

Secret Key #1 – Plan Big, Study Small

There's a lot riding on your performance. If you want to ace this test, you're going to need to keep your skills sharp and the material fresh in your mind. You need a plan that lets you review everything you need to know while still fitting in your schedule. We'll break this strategy down into three categories.

Information Organization

Start with the information you already have: the official test outline. From this, you can make a complete list of all the concepts you need to cover before the test. Organize these concepts into groups that can be studied together, and create a list of any related vocabulary you need to learn so you can brush up on any difficult terms. You'll want to keep this vocabulary list handy once you actually start studying since you may need to add to it along the way.

Time Management

Once you have your set of study concepts, decide how to spread them out over the time you have left before the test. Break your study plan into small, clear goals so you have a manageable task for each day and know exactly what you're doing. Then just focus on one small step at a time. When you manage your time this way, you don't need to spend hours at a time studying. Studying a small block of content for a short period each day helps you retain information better and avoid stressing over how much you have left to do. You can relax knowing that you have a plan to cover everything in time. In order for this strategy to be effective though, you have to start studying early and stick to your schedule. Avoid the exhaustion and futility that comes from last-minute cramming!

Study Environment

The environment you study in has a big impact on your learning. Studying in a coffee shop, while probably more enjoyable, is not likely to be as fruitful as studying in a quiet room. It's important to keep distractions to a minimum. You're only planning to study for a short block of time, so make the most of it. Don't pause to check your phone or get up to find a snack. It's also important to **avoid multitasking**. Research has consistently shown that multitasking will make your studying dramatically less effective. Your study area should also be comfortable and well-lit so you don't have the distraction of straining your eyes or sitting on an uncomfortable chair.

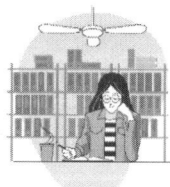 The time of day you study is also important. You want to be rested and alert. Don't wait until just before bedtime. Study when you'll be most likely to comprehend and remember. Even better, if you know what time of day your test will be, set that time aside for study. That way your brain will be used to working on that subject at that specific time and you'll have a better chance of recalling information.

Finally, it can be helpful to team up with others who are studying for the same test. Your actual studying should be done in as isolated an environment as possible, but the work of organizing the information and setting up the study plan can be divided up. In between study sessions, you can discuss with your teammates the concepts that you're all studying and quiz each other on the details. Just be sure that your teammates are as serious about the test as you are. If you find that your study time is being replaced with social time, you might need to find a new team.

2

Secret Key #2 – Make Your Studying Count

You're devoting a lot of time and effort to preparing for this test, so you want to be absolutely certain it will pay off. This means doing more than just reading the content and hoping you can remember it on test day. It's important to make every minute of study count. There are two main areas you can focus on to make your studying count.

Retention

It doesn't matter how much time you study if you can't remember the material. You need to make sure you are retaining the concepts. To check your retention of the information you're learning, try recalling it at later times with minimal prompting. Try carrying around flashcards and glance at one or two from time to time or ask a friend who's also studying for the test to quiz you.

To enhance your retention, look for ways to put the information into practice so that you can apply it rather than simply recalling it. If you're using the information in practical ways, it will be much easier to remember. Similarly, it helps to solidify a concept in your mind if you're not only reading it to yourself but also explaining it to someone else. Ask a friend to let you teach them about a concept you're a little shaky on (or speak aloud to an imaginary audience if necessary). As you try to summarize, define, give examples, and answer your friend's questions, you'll understand the concepts better and they will stay with you longer. Finally, step back for a big picture view and ask yourself how each piece of information fits with the whole subject. When you link the different concepts together and see them working together as a whole, it's easier to remember the individual components.

Finally, practice showing your work on any multi-step problems, even if you're just studying. Writing out each step you take to solve a problem will help solidify the process in your mind, and you'll be more likely to remember it during the test.

Modality

Modality simply refers to the means or method by which you study. Choosing a study modality that fits your own individual learning style is crucial. No two people learn best in exactly the same way, so it's important to know your strengths and use them to your advantage.

For example, if you learn best by visualization, focus on visualizing a concept in your mind and draw an image or a diagram. Try color-coding your notes, illustrating them, or creating symbols that will trigger your mind to recall a learned concept. If you learn best by hearing or discussing information, find a study partner who learns the same way or read aloud to yourself. Think about how to put the information in your own words. Imagine that you are giving a lecture on the topic and record yourself so you can listen to it later.

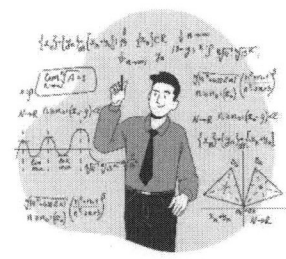

For any learning style, flashcards can be helpful. Organize the information so you can take advantage of spare moments to review. Underline key words or phrases. Use different colors for different categories. Mnemonic devices (such as creating a short list in which every item starts with the same letter) can also help with retention. Find what works best for you and use it to store the information in your mind most effectively and easily.

Secret Key #3 – Practice the Right Way

Your success on test day depends not only on how many hours you put into preparing, but also on whether you prepared the right way. It's good to check along the way to see if your studying is paying off. One of the most effective ways to do this is by taking practice tests to evaluate your progress. Practice tests are useful because they show exactly where you need to improve. Every time you take a practice test, pay special attention to these three groups of questions:

- The questions you got wrong
- The questions you had to guess on, even if you guessed right
- The questions you found difficult or slow to work through

This will show you exactly what your weak areas are, and where you need to devote more study time. Ask yourself why each of these questions gave you trouble. Was it because you didn't understand the material? Was it because you didn't remember the vocabulary? Do you need more repetitions on this type of question to build speed and confidence? Dig into those questions and figure out how you can strengthen your weak areas as you go back to review the material.

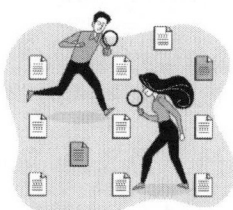 Additionally, many practice tests have a section explaining the answer choices. It can be tempting to read the explanation and think that you now have a good understanding of the concept. However, an explanation likely only covers part of the question's broader context. Even if the explanation makes perfect sense, **go back and investigate** every concept related to the question until you're positive you have a thorough understanding.

As you go along, keep in mind that the practice test is just that: practice. Memorizing these questions and answers will not be very helpful on the actual test because it is unlikely to have any of the same exact questions. If you only know the right answers to the sample questions, you won't be prepared for the real thing. **Study the concepts** until you understand them fully, and then you'll be able to answer any question that shows up on the test.

It's important to wait on the practice tests until you're ready. If you take a test on your first day of study, you may be overwhelmed by the amount of material covered and how much you need to learn. Work up to it gradually.

On test day, you'll need to be prepared for answering questions, managing your time, and using the test-taking strategies you've learned. It's a lot to balance, like a mental marathon that will have a big impact on your future. Like training for a marathon, you'll need to start slowly and work your way up. When test day arrives, you'll be ready.

Start with the strategies you've read in the first two Secret Keys—plan your course and study in the way that works best for you. If you have time, consider using multiple study resources to get different approaches to the same concepts. It can be helpful to see difficult concepts from more than one angle. Then find a good source for practice tests. Many times, the test website will suggest potential study resources or provide sample tests.

4

Practice Test Strategy

If you're able to find at least three practice tests, we recommend this strategy:

UNTIMED AND OPEN-BOOK PRACTICE

Take the first test with no time constraints and with your notes and study guide handy. Take your time and focus on applying the strategies you've learned.

TIMED AND OPEN-BOOK PRACTICE

Take the second practice test open-book as well, but set a timer and practice pacing yourself to finish in time.

TIMED AND CLOSED-BOOK PRACTICE

Take any other practice tests as if it were test day. Set a timer and put away your study materials. Sit at a table or desk in a quiet room, imagine yourself at the testing center, and answer questions as quickly and accurately as possible.

Keep repeating timed and closed-book tests on a regular basis until you run out of practice tests or it's time for the actual test. Your mind will be ready for the schedule and stress of test day, and you'll be able to focus on recalling the material you've learned.

Secret Key #4 – Pace Yourself

Once you're fully prepared for the material on the test, your biggest challenge on test day will be managing your time. Just knowing that the clock is ticking can make you panic even if you have plenty of time left. Work on pacing yourself so you can build confidence against the time constraints of the exam. Pacing is a difficult skill to master, especially in a high-pressure environment, so **practice is vital**.

Set time expectations for your pace based on how much time is available. For example, if a section has 60 questions and the time limit is 30 minutes, you know you have to average 30 seconds or less per question in order to answer them all. Although 30 seconds is the hard limit, set 25 seconds per question as your goal, so you reserve extra time to spend on harder questions. When you budget extra time for the harder questions, you no longer have any reason to stress when those questions take longer to answer.

Don't let this time expectation distract you from working through the test at a calm, steady pace, but keep it in mind so you don't spend too much time on any one question. Recognize that taking extra time on one question you don't understand may keep you from answering two that you do understand later in the test. If your time limit for a question is up and you're still not sure of the answer, mark it and move on, and come back to it later if the time and the test format allow. If the testing format doesn't allow you to return to earlier questions, just make an educated guess; then put it out of your mind and move on.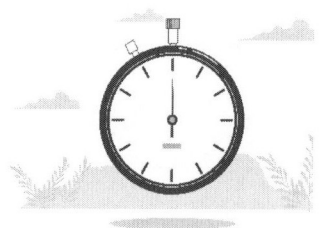

On the easier questions, be careful not to rush. It may seem wise to hurry through them so you have more time for the challenging ones, but it's not worth missing one if you know the concept and just didn't take the time to read the question fully. Work efficiently but make sure you understand the question and have looked at all of the answer choices, since more than one may seem right at first.

Even if you're paying attention to the time, you may find yourself a little behind at some point. You should speed up to get back on track, but do so wisely. Don't panic; just take a few seconds less on each question until you're caught up. Don't guess without thinking, but do look through the answer choices and eliminate any you know are wrong. If you can get down to two choices, it is often worthwhile to guess from those. Once you've chosen an answer, move on and don't dwell on any that you skipped or had to hurry through. If a question was taking too long, chances are it was one of the harder ones, so you weren't as likely to get it right anyway.

On the other hand, if you find yourself getting ahead of schedule, it may be beneficial to slow down a little. The more quickly you work, the more likely you are to make a careless mistake that will affect your score. You've budgeted time for each question, so don't be afraid to spend that time. Practice an efficient but careful pace to get the most out of the time you have.

6

Secret Key #5 – Have a Plan for Guessing

When you're taking the test, you may find yourself stuck on a question. Some of the answer choices seem better than others, but you don't see the one answer choice that is obviously correct. What do you do?

The scenario described above is very common, yet most test takers have not effectively prepared for it. Developing and practicing a plan for guessing may be one of the single most effective uses of your time as you get ready for the exam.

In developing your plan for guessing, there are three questions to address:

- When should you start the guessing process?
- How should you narrow down the choices?
- Which answer should you choose?

When to Start the Guessing Process

Unless your plan for guessing is to select C every time (which, despite its merits, is not what we recommend), you need to leave yourself enough time to apply your answer elimination strategies. Since you have a limited amount of time for each question, that means that if you're going to give yourself the best shot at guessing correctly, you have to decide quickly whether or not you will guess.

Of course, the best-case scenario is that you don't have to guess at all, so first, see if you can answer the question based on your knowledge of the subject and basic reasoning skills. Focus on the key words in the question and try to jog your memory of related topics. Give yourself a chance to bring the knowledge to mind, but once you realize that you don't have (or you can't access) the knowledge you need to answer the question, it's time to start the guessing process.

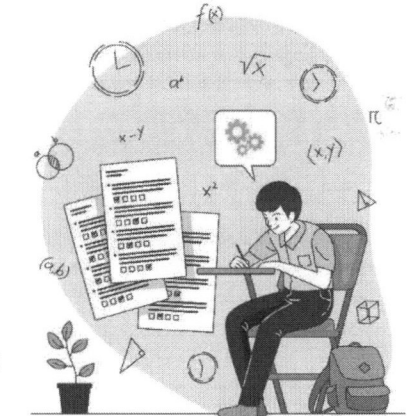

It's almost always better to start the guessing process too early than too late. It only takes a few seconds to remember something and answer the question from knowledge. Carefully eliminating wrong answer choices takes longer. Plus, going through the process of eliminating answer choices can actually help jog your memory.

Summary: Start the guessing process as soon as you decide that you can't answer the question based on your knowledge.

7

How to Narrow Down the Choices

The next chapter in this book (**Test-Taking Strategies**) includes a wide range of strategies for how to approach questions and how to look for answer choices to eliminate. You will definitely want to read those carefully, practice them, and figure out which ones work best for you. Here though, we're going to address a mindset rather than a particular strategy.

Your odds of guessing an answer correctly depend on how many options you are choosing from.

Number of options left	5	4	3	2	1
Odds of guessing correctly	20%	25%	33%	50%	100%

You can see from this chart just how valuable it is to be able to eliminate incorrect answers and make an educated guess, but there are two things that many test takers do that cause them to miss out on the benefits of guessing:

- Accidentally eliminating the correct answer
- Selecting an answer based on an impression

We'll look at the first one here, and the second one in the next section.

To avoid accidentally eliminating the correct answer, we recommend a thought exercise called **the $5 challenge**. In this challenge, you only eliminate an answer choice from contention if you are willing to bet $5 on it being wrong. Why $5? Five dollars is a small but not insignificant amount of money. It's an amount you could afford to lose but wouldn't want to throw away. And while losing

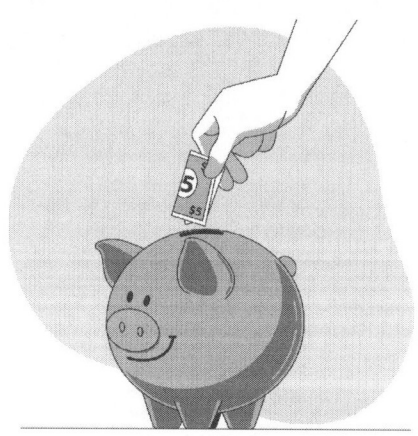

$5 once might not hurt too much, doing it twenty times will set you back $100. In the same way, each small decision you make—eliminating a choice here, guessing on a question there—won't by itself impact your score very much, but when you put them all together, they can make a big difference. By holding each answer choice elimination decision to a higher standard, you can reduce the risk of accidentally eliminating the correct answer.

The $5 challenge can also be applied in a positive sense: If you are willing to bet $5 that an answer choice *is* correct, go ahead and mark it as correct.

Summary: Only eliminate an answer choice if you are willing to bet $5 that it is wrong.

8

Which Answer to Choose

You're taking the test. You've run into a hard question and decided you'll have to guess. You've eliminated all the answer choices you're willing to bet $5 on. Now you have to pick an answer. Why do we even need to talk about this? Why can't you just pick whichever one you feel like when the time comes?

The answer to these questions is that if you don't come into the test with a plan, you'll rely on your impression to select an answer choice, and if you do that, you risk falling into a trap. The test writers know that everyone who takes their test will be guessing on some of the questions, so they intentionally write wrong answer choices to seem plausible. You still have to pick an answer though, and if the wrong answer choices are designed to look right, how can you ever be sure that you're not falling for their trap? The best solution we've found to this dilemma is to take the decision out of your hands entirely. Here is the process we recommend:

Once you've eliminated any choices that you are confident (willing to bet $5) are wrong, select the first remaining choice as your answer.

Whether you choose to select the first remaining choice, the second, or the last, the important thing is that you use some preselected standard. Using this approach guarantees that you will not be enticed into selecting an answer choice that looks right, because you are not basing your decision on how the answer choices look.

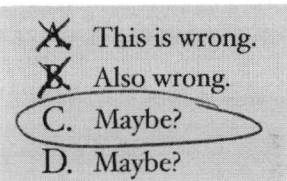

This is not meant to make you question your knowledge. Instead, it is to help you recognize the difference between your knowledge and your impressions. There's a huge difference between thinking an answer is right because of what you know, and thinking an answer is right because it looks or sounds like it should be right.

Summary: To ensure that your selection is appropriately random, make a predetermined selection from among all answer choices you have not eliminated.

Test-Taking Strategies

This section contains a list of test-taking strategies that you may find helpful as you work through the test. By taking what you know and applying logical thought, you can maximize your chances of answering any question correctly!

It is very important to realize that every question is different and every person is different: no single strategy will work on every question, and no single strategy will work for every person. That's why we've included all of them here, so you can try them out and determine which ones work best for different types of questions and which ones work best for you.

Question Strategies

⊘ READ CAREFULLY

Read the question and the answer choices carefully. Don't miss the question because you misread the terms. You have plenty of time to read each question thoroughly and make sure you understand what is being asked. Yet a happy medium must be attained, so don't waste too much time. You must read carefully and efficiently.

⊘ CONTEXTUAL CLUES

Look for contextual clues. If the question includes a word you are not familiar with, look at the immediate context for some indication of what the word might mean. Contextual clues can often give you all the information you need to decipher the meaning of an unfamiliar word. Even if you can't determine the meaning, you may be able to narrow down the possibilities enough to make a solid guess at the answer to the question.

⊘ PREFIXES

If you're having trouble with a word in the question or answer choices, try dissecting it. Take advantage of every clue that the word might include. Prefixes can be a huge help. Usually, they allow you to determine a basic meaning. *Pre-* means before, *post-* means after, *pro-* is positive, *de-* is negative. From prefixes, you can get an idea of the general meaning of the word and try to put it into context.

⊘ HEDGE WORDS

Watch out for critical hedge words, such as *likely, may, can, often, almost, mostly, usually, generally, rarely,* and *sometimes*. Question writers insert these hedge phrases to cover every possibility. Often an answer choice will be wrong simply because it leaves no room for exception. Be on guard for answer choices that have definitive words such as *exactly* and *always*.

⊘ SWITCHBACK WORDS

Stay alert for *switchbacks*. These are the words and phrases frequently used to alert you to shifts in thought. The most common switchback words are *but, although,* and *however*. Others include *nevertheless, on the other hand, even though, while, in spite of, despite,* and *regardless of*. Switchback words are important to catch because they can change the direction of the question or an answer choice.

⊘ Face Value

When in doubt, use common sense. Accept the situation in the problem at face value. Don't read too much into it. These problems will not require you to make wild assumptions. If you have to go beyond creativity and warp time or space in order to have an answer choice fit the question, then you should move on and consider the other answer choices. These are normal problems rooted in reality. The applicable relationship or explanation may not be readily apparent, but it is there for you to figure out. Use your common sense to interpret anything that isn't clear.

Answer Choice Strategies

⊘ Answer Selection

The most thorough way to pick an answer choice is to identify and eliminate wrong answers until only one is left, then confirm it is the correct answer. Sometimes an answer choice may immediately seem right, but be careful. The test writers will usually put more than one reasonable answer choice on each question, so take a second to read all of them and make sure that the other choices are not equally obvious. As long as you have time left, it is better to read every answer choice than to pick the first one that looks right without checking the others.

⊘ Answer Choice Families

An answer choice family consists of two (in rare cases, three) answer choices that are very similar in construction and cannot all be true at the same time. If you see two answer choices that are direct opposites or parallels, one of them is usually the correct answer. For instance, if one answer choice says that quantity x increases and another either says that quantity x decreases (opposite) or says that quantity y increases (parallel), then those answer choices would fall into the same family. An answer choice that doesn't match the construction of the answer choice family is more likely to be incorrect. Most questions will not have answer choice families, but when they do appear, you should be prepared to recognize them.

⊘ Eliminate Answers

Eliminate answer choices as soon as you realize they are wrong, but make sure you consider all possibilities. If you are eliminating answer choices and realize that the last one you are left with is also wrong, don't panic. Start over and consider each choice again. There may be something you missed the first time that you will realize on the second pass.

⊘ Avoid Fact Traps

Don't be distracted by an answer choice that is factually true but doesn't answer the question. You are looking for the choice that answers the question. Stay focused on what the question is asking for so you don't accidentally pick an answer that is true but incorrect. Always go back to the question and make sure the answer choice you've selected actually answers the question and is not merely a true statement.

⊘ Extreme Statements

In general, you should avoid answers that put forth extreme actions as standard practice or proclaim controversial ideas as established fact. An answer choice that states the "process should be used in certain situations, if…" is much more likely to be correct than one that states the "process should be discontinued completely." The first is a calm rational statement and doesn't even make a definitive, uncompromising stance, using a hedge word *if* to provide wiggle room, whereas the second choice is far more extreme.

⊘ Benchmark

As you read through the answer choices and you come across one that seems to answer the question well, mentally select that answer choice. This is not your final answer, but it's the one that will help you evaluate the other answer choices. The one that you selected is your benchmark or standard for judging each of the other answer choices. Every other answer choice must be compared to your benchmark. That choice is correct until proven otherwise by another answer choice beating it. If you find a better answer, then that one becomes your new benchmark. Once you've decided that no other choice answers the question as well as your benchmark, you have your final answer.

⊘ Predict the Answer

Before you even start looking at the answer choices, it is often best to try to predict the answer. When you come up with the answer on your own, it is easier to avoid distractions and traps because you will know exactly what to look for. The right answer choice is unlikely to be word-for-word what you came up with, but it should be a close match. Even if you are confident that you have the right answer, you should still take the time to read each option before moving on.

General Strategies

⊘ Tough Questions

If you are stumped on a problem or it appears too hard or too difficult, don't waste time. Move on! Remember though, if you can quickly check for obviously incorrect answer choices, your chances of guessing correctly are greatly improved. Before you completely give up, at least try to knock out a couple of possible answers. Eliminate what you can and then guess at the remaining answer choices before moving on.

⊘ Check Your Work

Since you will probably not know every term listed and the answer to every question, it is important that you get credit for the ones that you do know. Don't miss any questions through careless mistakes. If at all possible, try to take a second to look back over your answer selection and make sure you've selected the correct answer choice and haven't made a costly careless mistake (such as marking an answer choice that you didn't mean to mark). This quick double check should more than pay for itself in caught mistakes for the time it costs.

⊘ Pace Yourself

It's easy to be overwhelmed when you're looking at a page full of questions; your mind is confused and full of random thoughts, and the clock is ticking down faster than you would like. Calm down and maintain the pace that you have set for yourself. Especially as you get down to the last few minutes of the test, don't let the small numbers on the clock make you panic. As long as you are on track by monitoring your pace, you are guaranteed to have time for each question.

⊘ Don't Rush

It is very easy to make errors when you are in a hurry. Maintaining a fast pace in answering questions is pointless if it makes you miss questions that you would have gotten right otherwise. Test writers like to include distracting information and wrong answers that seem right. Taking a little extra time to avoid careless mistakes can make all the difference in your test score. Find a pace that allows you to be confident in the answers that you select.

⊘ Keep Moving

Panicking will not help you pass the test, so do your best to stay calm and keep moving. Taking deep breaths and going through the answer elimination steps you practiced can help to break through a stress barrier and keep your pace.

Final Notes

The combination of a solid foundation of content knowledge and the confidence that comes from practicing your plan for applying that knowledge is the key to maximizing your performance on test day. As your foundation of content knowledge is built up and strengthened, you'll find that the strategies included in this chapter become more and more effective in helping you quickly sift through the distractions and traps of the test to isolate the correct answer.

Now that you're preparing to move forward into the test content chapters of this book, be sure to keep your goal in mind. As you read, think about how you will be able to apply this information on the test. If you've already seen sample questions for the test and you have an idea of the question format and style, try to come up with questions of your own that you can answer based on what you're reading. This will give you valuable practice applying your knowledge in the same ways you can expect to on test day.

Good luck and good studying!

14

Cardiovascular Patient Care Problems

Cardiac Conditions

ACUTE CORONARY SYNDROMES

Acute coronary syndrome (ACS) is the impairment of blood flow through the coronary arteries, leading to ischemia of the cardiac muscle. Angina frequently occurs in ACS, manifesting as crushing pain substernally, radiating down the left arm or both arms. However, in females, elderly, and diabetics, symptoms may appear less acute and include nausea, shortness of breath, fatigue, pain/weakness/numbness in arms, or no pain at all (*silent ischemia*). There are multiple **classifications of angina**:

- **Stable angina**: Exercise-induced, short lived, relieved by rest or nitroglycerin. Other precipitating events include decrease in environmental temperature, heavy eating, strong emotions (such as fright or anger), or exertion, including coitus.
- **Unstable angina** (preinfarction or crescendo angina): A change in the pattern of stable angina, characterized by an increase in pain, not responding to a single nitroglycerin or rest, and persisting for >5 minutes. May cause a change in EKG, or indicate rupture of an atherosclerotic plaque or the beginning of thrombus formation. Treat as a medical emergency, indicates impending MI.
- **Variant angina** (Prinzmetal's angina): Results from spasms of the coronary arteries. Associated with or without atherosclerotic plaques and is often related to smoking, alcohol, or illicit stimulants, but can occur cyclically and at rest. Elevation of ST segments usually occurs with variant angina. Treatment is nitroglycerin or calcium channel blockers.

> **Review Video: Coronary Artery Disease**
> Visit mometrix.com/academy and enter code: 950720

MYOCARDIAL INFARCTIONS
NSTEMI AND *STEMI*

Non–ST-segment elevation MI (NSTEMI): ST elevation on the electrocardiogram (ECG) occurs in response to myocardial damage resulting from infarction or severe ischemia. The absence of ST elevation may be diagnosed as unstable angina or NSTEMI, but cardiac enzyme levels increase with NSTEMI, indicating partial blockage of coronary arteries with some damage. Symptoms are consistent with unstable angina, with chest pain or tightness, pain radiating to the neck or arm, dyspnea, anxiety, weakness, dizziness, nausea, vomiting, and heartburn. Initial treatment may include nitroglycerin, β-blockers, antiplatelet agents, or antithrombotic agents. Ongoing treatment may include β-blockers, aspirin, statins, angiotensin-converting enzyme inhibitors, angiotensin-receptor blockers, and clopidogrel. Percutaneous coronary intervention is not recommended.

ST-segment elevation MI (STEMI): This more severe type of MI involves complete blockage of one or more coronary arteries with myocardial damage, resulting in ST elevation. Symptoms are those of acute MI. As necrosis occurs, Q waves often develop, indicating irreversible myocardial damage, which may result in death, so treatment involves immediate reperfusion before necrosis can occur.

> **Review Video: Myocardial Infarction**
> Visit mometrix.com/academy and enter code: 148923

Q-WAVE AND NON-Q-WAVE MYOCARDIAL INFARCTIONS

Formerly classified as transmural or non-transmural, myocardial infarctions are now classified as Q-wave or non-Q-wave:

- **Q-Wave**
  - Characterized by a series of abnormal Q waves (wider and deeper) on ECG, especially in the early morning (related to adrenergic activity).
  - Infarction is usually prolonged and results in necrosis.
  - Coronary occlusion is complete in 80-90% of cases.
  - Q-wave MI is often, but not always, transmural.
  - Peak CK levels occur in about 27 hours.
- **Non-Q-Wave**
  - Characterized by changes in ST-T wave with ST depression (usually reversible within a few days).
  - Usually reperfusion occurs spontaneously, so infarct size is smaller. Contraction necrosis related to reperfusion is common.
  - Non-Q-wave MI is usually non-transmural.
  - Coronary occlusion is complete in only 20-30%.
  - Peak CK levels occur in 12-13 hours.
  - Reinfarction is common.

LOCATIONS AND TYPES

Myocardial infarctions are also classified according to their location and the extent of injury. Q-wave infarctions involve the full thickness of the heart muscle, often producing a series of Q waves on ECG. While an MI most frequently damages the left ventricle and the septum, the right ventricle may be damaged as well, depending upon the area of the occlusion:

- **Anterior** (V_2 to V_4): Occlusion in the proximal left anterior descending (LAD) or left coronary artery. Reciprocal changes found in leads II, III, aV_F.
- **Lateral** (I, aV_L, V_5, V_6): Occlusion of the circumflex coronary artery or branch of left coronary artery. Often causes damage to anterior wall as well. Reciprocal changes found in leads II, III, aV_F.
- **Inferior/diaphragmatic** (II, III, aV_F): Occlusion of the right coronary artery and causes conduction malfunctions. Reciprocal changes found in leads I and aV_L.
- **Right ventricular** (V_{4R}, V_{5R}, V_{6R}): Occlusion of the proximal section of the right coronary artery and damages in the right ventricle and the inferior wall. No reciprocal changes should be noted on an ECG.
- **Posterior** (V_8, V_9): Occlusion in the right coronary artery or circumflex artery and may be difficult to diagnose. Reciprocal changes found in V_1-V_4.

CLINICAL MANIFESTATIONS AND DIAGNOSIS

Clinical manifestations of myocardial infarction may vary considerably. More than half of all patients present with acute MIs with no prior history of cardiovascular disease.

Signs/symptoms: Angina with pain in chest that may radiate to neck or arms, palpitations, hypertension or hypotension, dyspnea, pulmonary edema, dependent edema, nausea/vomiting, pallor, skin cold and clammy, diaphoresis, decreased urinary output, neurological/psychological disturbances: anxiety, light-headedness, headache, visual abnormalities, slurred speech, and fear.

Diagnosis is based on the following:

- ECG obtained immediately to monitor heart changes over time. Typical changes include T-wave inversion, elevation of ST segment, abnormal Q waves, tachycardia, bradycardia, and dysrhythmias.
- Echocardiogram: decreased ventricular function is possible, especially for transmural MI.
- Labs:
  - **Troponin**: Increases within 3–6 hours, peaks 14–20; elevated for up to 1-2 weeks.
  - **Creatinine kinase (CK-MB)**: Increases 4–8 hours and peaks at about 24 hours (earlier with thrombolytic therapy or PTCA).
  - **Ischemia Modified Albumin (IMA)**: Increase within minutes, peak 6 hours and return to baseline; verify with other labs.
  - **Myoglobin**: Increases in 0.5–4.0 hours, peaks 6–7 hours. While an increase is not specific to an MI, a failure to increase can be used to rule out an MI.

CARDIAC TAMPONADE

Cardiac tamponade occurs with pericardial effusion, causing pressure against the heart. It may be a complication of trauma, pericarditis, cardiac surgery, pneumothorax, or heart failure. About 50 mL of fluid normally circulates in the pericardial area to reduce friction, and a sudden increase in this volume or air in the pericardial sac can compress the heart, causing a number of cardiac responses such as:

- Increased end-diastolic pressure in both ventricles
- Decrease in venous return
- Decrease in ventricular filling

Symptoms may include pressure or pain in the chest, dyspnea, and pulsus paradoxus >10 mmHg. Beck's triad (increased CVP, distended neck veins, muffled heart sounds, and hypotension) is common. A sudden decrease in chest tube drainage can occur as fluid and clots accumulate in the pericardial sac, preventing the blood from filling the ventricles and decreasing cardiac output and perfusion of the body, including the kidneys (resulting in decreased urinary output). X-ray may show change in cardiac silhouette and mediastinal shift (in 20%). Treatment includes pericardiocentesis with large bore needle or surgical repair to control bleeding and relieve cardiac compression. Risk factors include cardiac surgery, cardiac tumors, MI, and chest trauma.

> **Review Video: Cardiac Tamponade**
> Visit mometrix.com/academy and enter code: 920182

CARDIOMYOPATHY

DILATED CARDIOMYOPATHY

Dilated cardiomyopathy (DCM) occurs when some precipitating factor leads to decreased cardiac perfusion. The resulting ischemic cardiac tissue is replaced with scar tissue, and the healthy cells are forced to over-compensate, causing hypertrophy and over stretching. Eventually, the muscle cells become stretched beyond compensation, and dilated and weak chamber results, unable to properly contract. This causes a decrease in stroke volume and cardiac output, with the end result being enlargement of the mitral and tricuspid valves and severe valve regurgitation. While DCM is the most common form of cardiomyopathy, causes include:

- **Vascular**: Cardiac ischemia, hypertension, atherosclerosis
- **Metabolic**: Diabetes, uremia, thyrotoxicosis, and acromegaly, muscular dystrophy

- **Genetics** (familial DCM), and childbirth (peripartum DCM)
- **Viral infections,** particularly adenovirus, Varicella zoster, HIV, and Hepatitis C may cause DCM
- **Alcohol poisoning or cocaine addiction**
- **Radiation or heavy metal poisoning**, specifically cobalt

Signs/Symptoms: Dyspnea, SOB, tachycardia, S3/S4 heart sounds, holosystolic murmur, wheezes/crackles, pleural effusions, edema, JVD, ascites

Diagnosis: EKG (tachycardia/T wave changes), chest x-ray (cardiomegaly), 2D Echocardiogram (valve regurgitation/EF).

Treatment includes:

- Treat underlying cause if possible; supportive care
- Heart transplant if patient is a candidate and damage is permanent

HYPERTROPHIC CARDIOMYOPATHY

Hypertrophic cardiomyopathy (HCM) is a genetic disorder that causes idiopathic thickening of the heart muscle, primarily involving the ventricular septum and portions of the left ventricle. Patients with HCM produce abnormal sarcomeres and misalignment of muscle cells (myocardial disarray). Basically, HCM is characterized by ventricular hypertrophy, an asymmetrical septum, forceful systole, cardiac dysrhythmias, and myocardial disarray. Because the abnormal cells develop over time, it is common for HCM to remain undiagnosed until middle or late adulthood.

Signs/Symptoms: Exertional or atypical chest pain, dyspnea at rest, syncope, frequent palpitations (common due to reoccurring dysrhythmias).

Diagnosis: 2D echo (structure and EF), EKG (pathological Q waves and dysrhythmias), x-ray (cardiomegaly), Family history (especially cardiac death, reoccurring dysrhythmias, or myocardial hypertrophy).

Treatment includes:

- **Surgery**: Septal myectomy is gold standard: high mortality (3-10%), but increases cardiac output and quality of life.
- **Alcohol-based septal ablation**: Ethanol 100% injected into a branch of the LAD, creating a controlled area of infarction and consequently thinning the septum.

RESTRICTIVE CARDIOMYOPATHY

Restrictive cardiomyopathy (RCM) occurs when the ventricles become stiff and noncompliant, resulting in decreased end-diastolic cardiac refill volume. The ventricular stiffening is caused by the infiltration of fibroelastic tissue into the cardiac muscle (such as in amyloidosis or sarcoidosis). Atrial enlargement can be seen in most cases of RCM as a result of the increased effort required to push blood from the atria into the ventricles. It is not uncommon for a patient to be in atrial fibrillation secondary to atrial enlargement. In advanced cases, ventricular dysrhythmias may also be seen.

Signs/Symptoms: Exercise intolerance/fatigue, edema, crackles, elevated CVP, S3/S4, murmur, SOB at rest

Diagnosis: 2D echo (enlarged atria, decreased compliance of ventricle), hemodynamic monitoring (increased right atrial pressure and pulmonary wedge pressure, and SVR), x-ray (cardiomegaly), EKG (atrial fibrillation), endomyocardial biopsy (to differentiate from constrictive pericarditis).

Treatment includes:

- **Medications**: β-blockers increase ventricular filling; antiarrhythmics may be ordered
- **Surgical**: Heart transplant, if patient is a candidate

DYSRHYTHMIAS

SINUS BRADYCARDIA

There are 3 primary types of **sinus node dysrhythmias**: sinus bradycardia, sinus tachycardia, and sinus arrhythmia. **Sinus bradycardia (SB)** is caused by a decreased rate of impulse from sinus node. The pulse and ECG usually appear normal except for a slower rate.

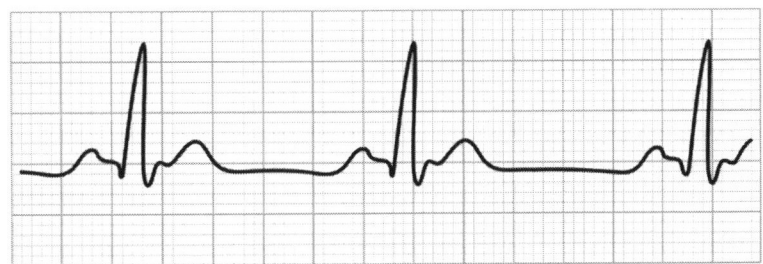

SB is characterized by a regular pulse <50-60 bpm with P waves in front of QRS, which are usually normal in shape and duration. PR interval is 0.12-0.20 seconds, QRS interval is 0.04-0.11 seconds, and P:QRS ratio of 1:1. SB may be caused by several factors:

- May be normal in athletes and older adults; generally not treated unless symptomatic
- Conditions that lower the body's metabolic needs, such as hypothermia or sleep
- Hypotension and decrease in oxygenation
- Medications such as calcium channel blockers and β-blockers
- Vagal stimulation that may result from vomiting, suctioning, defecating, or certain medical procedures (carotid stent placement, etc.)
- Increased intracranial pressure
- Myocardial infarction

Treatment: involves eliminating cause if possible, such as changing medications. Atropine 0.5-1.0 mg may be given IV to block vagal stimulation or increase rate if symptomatic.

SINUS TACHYCARDIA

Sinus tachycardia (ST) occurs when the sinus node impulse increases in frequency. ST is characterized by a regular pulse >100 with P waves before QRS but sometimes part of the

19

preceding T wave. QRS is usually of normal shape and duration (0.04-0.11 seconds) but may have consistent irregularity. PR interval is 0.12-0.20 seconds and P:QRS ratio of 1:1.

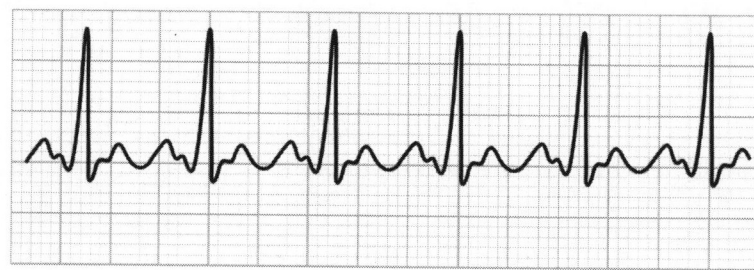

The rapid pulse decreases diastolic filling time and causes reduced cardiac output with resultant hypotension. Acute pulmonary edema may result from the decreased ventricular filling if untreated. ST may be **caused** by a number of factors:

- Acute blood loss, shock, hypovolemia, anemia
- Sinus arrhythmia, hypovolemic heart failure
- Hypermetabolic conditions, fever, infection
- Exertion/exercise, anxiety, stress
- Medications, such as sympathomimetic drugs

Treatment: eliminating precipitating factors, calcium channel blockers and β-blockers to reduce heart rate.

SUPRAVENTRICULAR TACHYCARDIA

Supraventricular tachycardia (SVT) (>100 BPM) may have a sudden onset and result in congestive heart failure. Rate may increase to 200–300 BPM, which will significantly decrease cardiac output due to decreased filling time. SVT originates in the atria rather than the ventricles but is controlled by the tissue in the area of the AV node rather than the SA node. Rhythm is usually rapid but regular. The P wave is present but may not be clearly defined as it may be obscured by the preceding T wave, and the QRS complex appears normal. The PR interval is 0.12-0.20 seconds and the QRS interval is 0.04-0.11 seconds with a P:QRS ratio of 1:1.

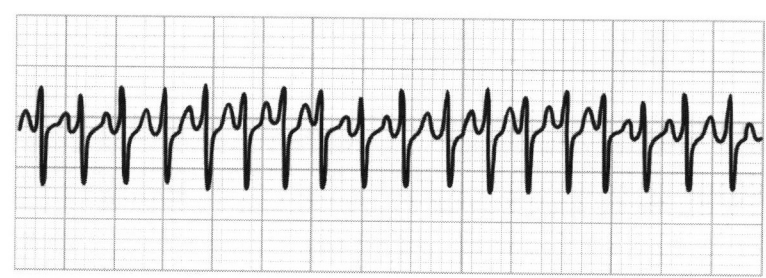

SVT may be episodic with periods of normal heart rate and rhythm between episodes of SVT, so it is often referred to as paroxysmal SVT (PSVT).

Treatment: Adenosine, digoxin (Lanoxin®), Verapamil (Calan®, Verelan®), vagal maneuvers, cardioversion.

SINUS ARRHYTHMIA

Sinus arrhythmia (SA) results from irregular impulses from the sinus node, often paradoxical (increasing with inspiration and decreasing with expiration) because of stimulation of the vagal nerve during inspiration and rarely causes a negative hemodynamic effect. These cyclic changes in the pulse during respiration are quite common in both children and young adults and often lesson with age but may persist in some adults. Sinus arrhythmia can, in some cases, relate to heart or valvular disease and may be increased with vagal stimulation for suctioning, vomiting, or defecating. Characteristics of SA include a regular pulse 50-100 BPM, P waves in front of QRS with duration (0.04-0.11 seconds) and shape of QRS usually normal, PR interval of 0.12-0.20 seconds, and P:QRS ratio of 1:1.

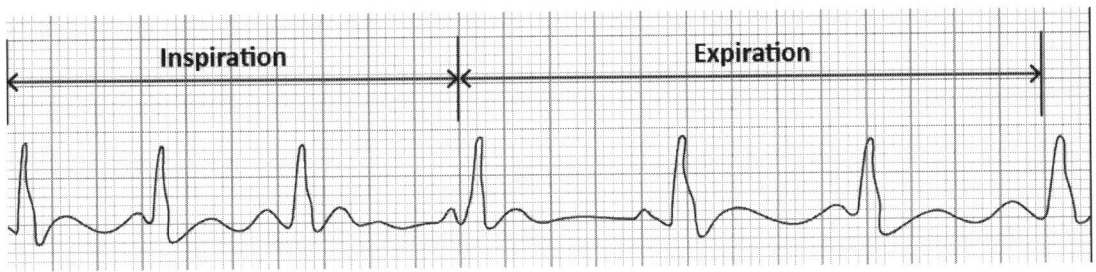

Treatment is usually not necessary unless it is associated with bradycardia.

PREMATURE ATRIAL CONTRACTION

There are 3 primary types of **atrial dysrhythmias**: premature atrial contraction, atrial flutter, and atrial fibrillation. Premature atrial contraction (PAC) is essentially an extra beat precipitated by an electrical impulse to the atrium before the sinus node impulse. The extra beat may be caused by alcohol, caffeine, nicotine, hypervolemia, hypokalemia, hypermetabolic conditions, atrial ischemia, or infarction. Characteristics include an irregular pulse because of extra P waves, the shape and duration of QRS is usually normal (0.04-0.11 seconds) but may be abnormal, PR interval remains between 0.12-0.20, and P:QRS ratio is 1:1. Rhythm is irregular with varying P-P and R-R intervals.

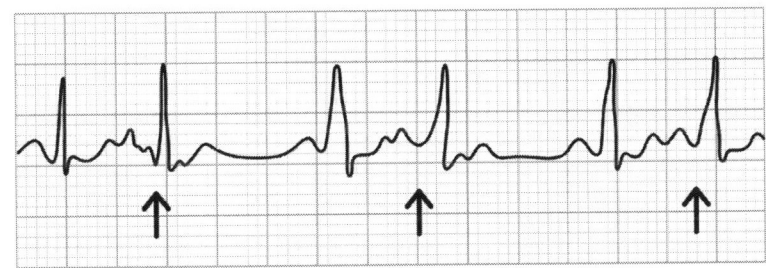

PACs can occur in an essentially healthy heart and are not usually cause for concern unless they are frequent (>6 per hr) and cause severe palpitations. In that case, atrial fibrillation should be suspected.

ATRIAL FLUTTER

Atrial flutter (AF) occurs when the atrial rate is faster, usually 250-400 beats per minute, than the AV node conduction rate so not all of the beats are conducted into the ventricles. The beats are effectively blocked at the AV node, preventing ventricular fibrillation although some extra ventricular impulses may pass through. AF is caused by the same conditions that cause A-fib: coronary artery disease, valvular disease, pulmonary disease, heavy alcohol ingestion, and cardiac surgery. AF is characterized by atrial rates of 250-400 with ventricular rates of 75-150, with ventricular rate usually being regular. P waves are saw-toothed (referred to as F waves), QRS shape and duration (0.04-0.11 seconds) are usually normal, PR interval may be hard to calculate because

21

of F waves, and the P:QRS ratio is 2:1 to 4:1. Symptoms include chest pain, dyspnea, and hypotension.

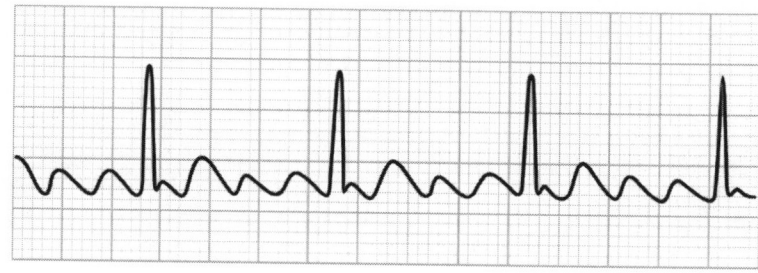

Treatment includes:

- Emergent cardioversion if condition is unstable
- Medications to slow ventricular rate and conduction through AV node: non-dihydropyridine calcium channel blockers (Cardizem®, Calan®) and beta blockers
- Medications to convert to sinus rhythm: Corvert®, Tikosyn, Amiodarone; also used in practice: Cardioquin®, Norpace®, Cordarone®

ATRIAL FIBRILLATION

Atrial fibrillation (A-fib) is rapid, disorganized atrial beats that are ineffective in emptying the atria, so that blood pools in the chambers. This can lead to thrombus formation and emboli. The ventricular rate increases with a decreased stroke volume, and cardiac output decreases with increased myocardial ischemia, resulting in palpitations and fatigue. A-fib is caused by coronary artery disease, valvular disease, pulmonary disease, heavy alcohol ingestion, infection, and cardiac surgery; however, it can also be idiopathic. A-fib is characterized by a very irregular pulse with atrial rate of 300-600 and ventricular rate of 120-200, shape and duration (0.04-0.11 seconds) of QRS is usually normal. Fibrillatory (F) waves are seen instead of P waves. The PR interval cannot be measured and the P:QRS ratio is highly variable.

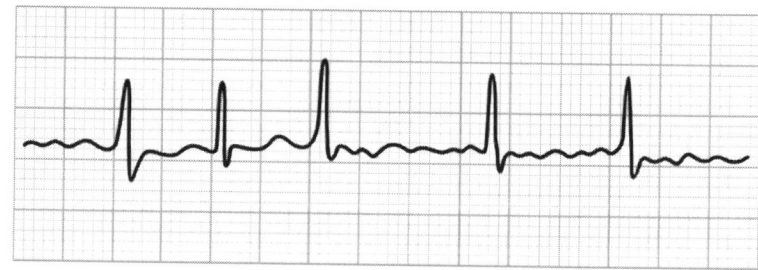

Treatment is the same as atrial flutter.

> **Review Video: Atrial Fibrillation and Atrial Flutter**
> Visit mometrix.com/academy and enter code: 263842

PREMATURE JUNCTIONAL CONTRACTION

The area around the AV node is the junction, and dysrhythmias that arise from that area are called junctional dysrhythmias. Premature junctional contraction (PJC) occurs when a premature impulse starts at the AV node before the next normal sinus impulse reaches the AV node. PJC is similar to premature atrial contraction (PAC) and generally requires no treatment although it may be an indication of digoxin toxicity. The ECG may appear basically normal with an early QRS complex that is normal in shape and duration (0.04-0.11 seconds). The P wave may be absent or it may precede,

22

be part of, or follow the QRS with a PR interval of 0.12 seconds. The P:QRS ratio may vary from <1:1 to 1:1 (with inverted P wave). The underlying rhythm is usually regular at a heart rate of 60-100. Significant symptoms related to PJC are rare.

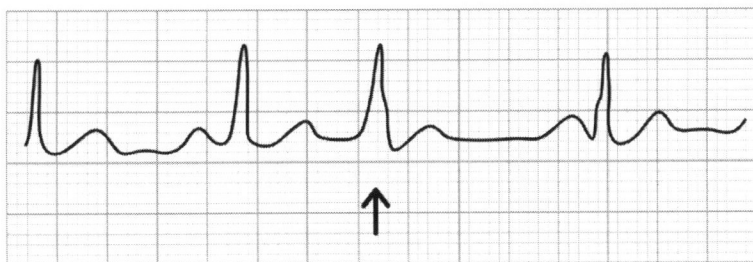

JUNCTIONAL RHYTHMS

Junctional rhythms occur when the AV node becomes the pacemaker of the heart. This can happen because the sinus node is depressed from increased vagal tone or a block at the AV node prevents sinus node impulses from being transmitted. While the sinus node normally sends impulses 60-100 beats per minute, the AV node junction usually sends impulses at 40-60 beats per minute. The QRS complex is of usual shape and duration (0.04-0.11 seconds). The P wave may be inverted and may be absent, hidden or after the QRS. If the P wave precedes the QRS, the PR interval is <0.12 seconds. The P:QRS ratio is <1:1 or 1:1. The junctional escape rhythm is a protective mechanism preventing asystole with failure of the sinus node. An **accelerated junctional rhythm** is similar, but the heart rate is 60-100. **Junctional tachycardia** occurs with heart rate of >100.

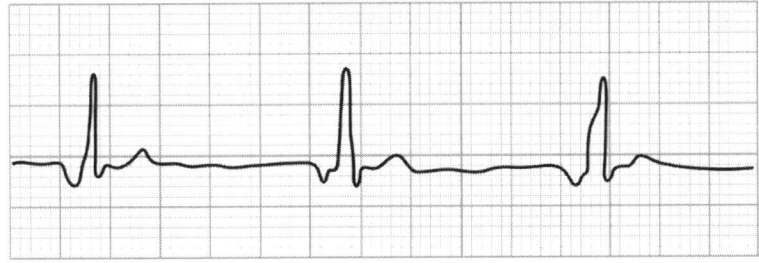

AV NODAL REENTRY TACHYCARDIA

AV nodal reentry tachycardia occurs when an impulse conducts to the area of the AV node and is then sent in a rapidly repeating cycle back to the same area and to the ventricles, resulting in a fast ventricular rate. The onset and cessation are usually rapid. AV nodal reentry tachycardia (also known as paroxysmal atrial tachycardia or supraventricular tachycardia if there are no P waves) is characterized by atrial rate of 150-250 with ventricular rate of 75-250, P wave that is difficult to see or absent, QRS complex that is usually normal and a PR interval of <0.12 if a P wave is present. The P:QRS ratio is 1-2:1. Precipitating factors include nicotine, caffeine, hypoxemia, anxiety, underlying coronary artery disease and cardiomyopathy. Cardiac output may be decreased with a rapid heart rate, causing dyspnea, chest pain, and hypotension.

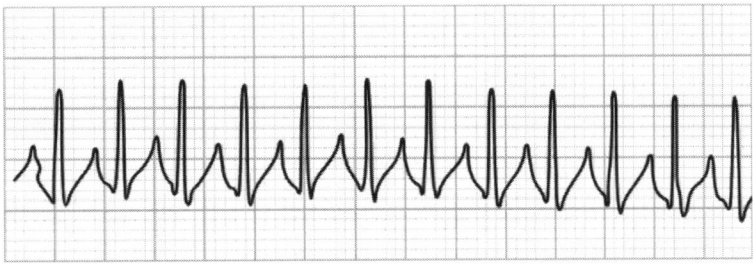

Treatment includes:

- Vagal maneuvers (carotid sinus massage, gag reflex, holding breath/bearing down)
- Medications (adenosine, verapamil, or diltiazem)
- Cardioversion if other methods unsuccessful

PREMATURE VENTRICULAR CONTRACTIONS

Premature ventricular contractions (PVCs) are those in which the impulse begins in the ventricles and conducts through them prior to the next sinus impulse. The ectopic QRS complexes may vary in shape, depending upon whether there is one site (unifocal) or more (multifocal) that stimulates the ectopic beats. PVCs usually cause no morbidity unless there is underlying cardiac disease or an acute MI. PVCs are characterized by an irregular heartbeat, QRS that is ≥0.12 seconds and oddly shaped. PVCs are often not treated in otherwise healthy people. PVCs may be precipitated by electrolyte imbalances, caffeine, nicotine, or alcohol. Because PVCs may occur with any supraventricular dysrhythmia, the underlying rhythm must be noted as well as the PVCs. If there are more than six PVCs in an hour, that is a risk factor for developing ventricular tachycardia.

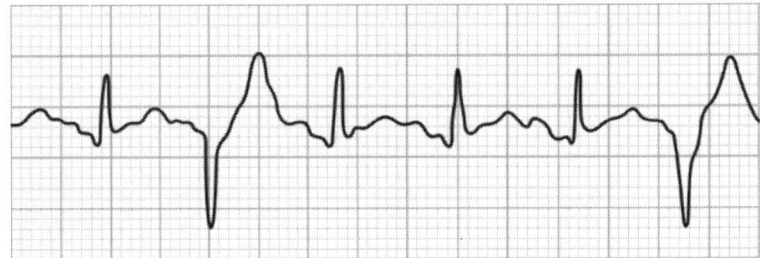

Bigeminy is a rhythm where every other beat is a PVC. **Trigeminy** is a rhythm where every third beat is a PVC.

Ventricular bigeminy is a rhythm where every other beat is a PVC. **Ventricular trigeminy** is a rhythm where every third beat is a PVC.

Treatment: Lidocaine (affects the ventricles, may cause CNS toxicity with nausea and vomiting), Procainamide (affects the atria and ventricles and may cause decreased BP and widening of QRS and QT); treat underlying cause.

VENTRICULAR TACHYCARDIA

Ventricular tachycardia (VT) is greater than 3 PVCs in a row with a ventricular rate of 100-200 beats per minute. Ventricular tachycardia may be triggered by the same factors as PVCs and often is related to underlying coronary artery disease. The rapid rate of contractions makes VT dangerous as the ineffective beats may render the person unconscious with no palpable pulse. A detectable rate is usually regular and the QRS complex is ≥0.12 seconds and is usually abnormally shaped. The

P wave may be undetectable with an irregular PR interval if P wave is present. The P:QRS ratio is often difficult to ascertain because of the absence of P waves.

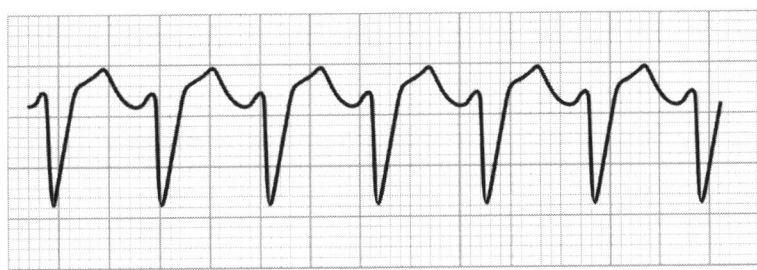

Treatment is as follows:

- With pulse: Synchronized cardioversion, adenosine
- No pulse: Same as ventricular fibrillation

NARROW COMPLEX AND WIDE COMPLEX TACHYCARDIAS

Tachycardias are classified as narrow complex or wide complex. Wide and narrow refer to the configuration of the QRS complex.

- **Wide complex tachycardia (WCT)**: About 80% of cases of WCT are caused by ventricular tachycardia. WCT originates at some point below the AV node and may be associated with palpitations, dyspnea, anxiety, diaphoresis, and cardiac arrest. Wide complex tachycardia is diagnosed with more than 3 consecutive beats at a heart rate >100 BPM and QRS duration ≥0.12 seconds.

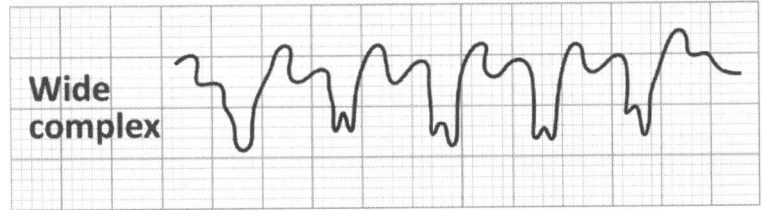

- **Narrow complex tachycardia (NCT)**: NCT is associated with palpitations, dyspnea, and peripheral edema. NCT is generally supraventricular in origin. Narrow complex tachycardia is diagnosed with ≥3 consecutive beats at heart rate of >100 BPM and QRS duration of <0.12 seconds.

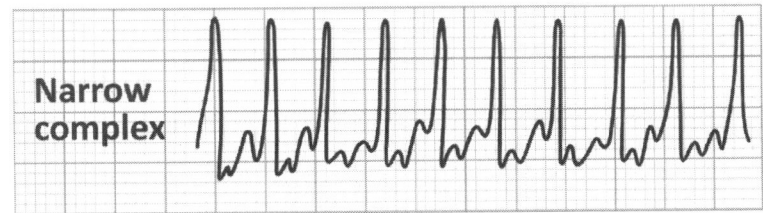

VENTRICULAR FIBRILLATION

Ventricular fibrillation (VF) is a rapid, very irregular ventricular rate >300 beats per minute with no atrial activity observable on the ECG, caused by disorganized electrical activity in the ventricles. The QRS complex is not recognizable as ECG shows irregular undulations. The causes are the same as for ventricular tachycardia and asystole. VF is accompanied by lack of palpable pulse, audible pulse, and respirations and is immediately life threatening without defibrillation.

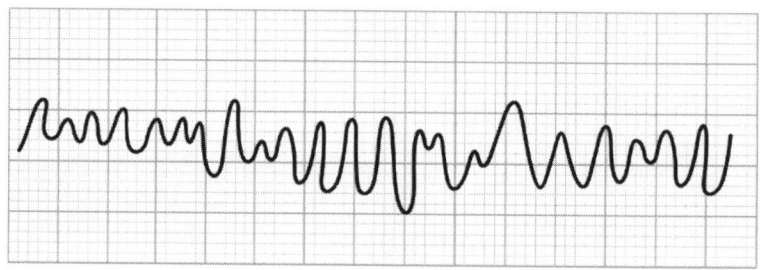

Treatment includes:

- Emergency defibrillation, the cause should be identified and treated
- Epinephrine 1 mg q 3-5minutes then amiodarone 300mg (2nd dose: 150mg) IV push

> **Review Video: Ventricular Arrythmias**
> Visit mometrix.com/academy and enter code: 933152

IDIOVENTRICULAR RHYTHM

Ventricular escape rhythm (idioventricular) occurs when the Purkinje fibers below the AV node create an impulse. This may occur if the sinus node fails to fire or if there is blockage at the AV node so that the impulse does not go through. Idioventricular rhythm is characterized by a regular ventricular rate of 20-40 BPM. Rates >40 BPM are called accelerated idioventricular rhythm. The P wave is missing and the QRS complex has a very bizarre and abnormal shape with duration of ≥0.12 seconds. The low ventricular rate may cause a decrease in cardiac output, often making the patient lose consciousness. In other patients, the idioventricular rhythm may not be associated with reduced cardiac output.

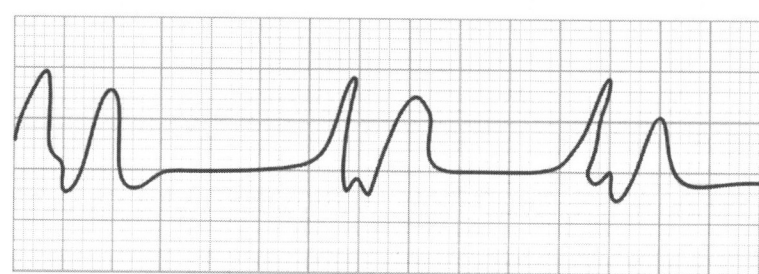

VENTRICULAR ASYSTOLE

Ventricular asystole is the absence of audible heartbeat, palpable pulse, and respirations, a condition often referred to as "cardiac arrest." While the ECG may show some P waves initially, the QRS complex is absent although there may be an occasional QRS "escape beat" (agonal rhythm). Cardiopulmonary resuscitation is required with intubation for ventilation and establishment of an intravenous line for fluids. Without immediate treatment, the patient will suffer from severe hypoxia and brain death within minutes. Identifying the cause is critical for the patient's survival. Consider the "Hs & Ts": hypovolemia, hypoxia, hydrogen ions (acidosis), hypo/hyperkalemia, hypothermia, tension pneumothorax, tamponade (cardiac), toxins, and thrombosis (pulmonary or coronary). Even with immediate treatment, the prognosis is poor and ventricular asystole is often a sign of impending death.

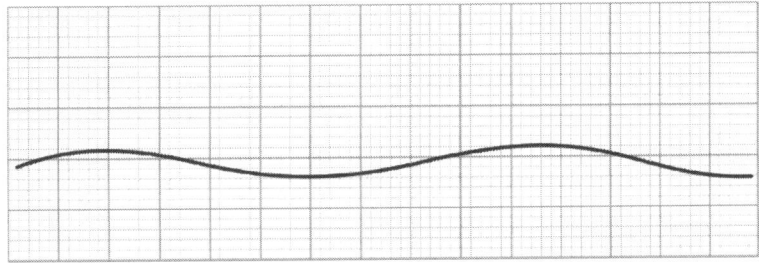

Treatment includes:

- CPR only; Asystole is not a shockable rhythm therefore defibrillation is not indicated
- Epinephrine 1 mg q 3-5 minutes

SINUS PAUSE

Sinus pause occurs when the sinus node fails to function properly to stimulate heart contractions, so there is a pause on the ECG recording that may persist for a few seconds to minutes, depending on the severity of the dysfunction. A prolonged pause may be difficult to differentiate from cardiac arrest. During the sinus pause, the P wave, QRS complex and PR and QRS intervals are all absent. P:QRS ratio is 1:1 and the rhythm is irregular. The pulse rate may vary widely, usually 60-100 BPM. Patients with frequent pauses may complain of dizziness or syncope. The patient may need to undergo an electrophysiology study and medication reconciliation to determine the cause. If measures such as decreasing medication are not effective, a pacemaker is usually indicated (if symptomatic).

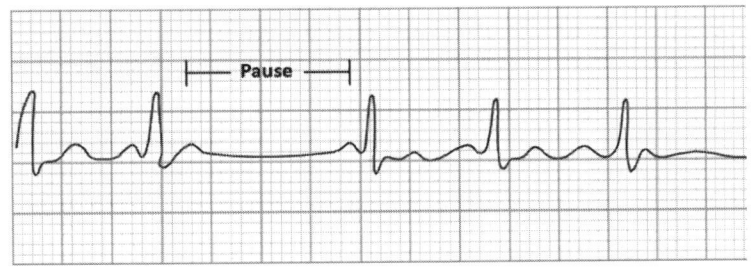

FIRST-DEGREE AV BLOCK

First-degree AV block occurs when the atrial impulses are conducted through the AV node to the ventricles at a rate that is slower than normal. While the P and QRS are usually normal, the PR interval is >0.20 seconds, and the P:QRS ratio is 1:1. A narrow QRS complex indicates a conduction abnormality only in the AV node, but a widened QRS indicates associated damage to the bundle branches as well. *Chronic* first-degree block may be caused by fibrosis/sclerosis of the conduction system related to coronary artery disease, valvular disease, cardiac myopathies and carries little morbidity, thus is often left untreated. *Acute* first-degree block, on the other hand, is of much more concern and may be related to digoxin toxicity, β-blockers, amiodarone, myocardial infarction, hyperkalemia, or edema related to valvular surgery.

Treatment: involves eliminating cause if possible, such as changing medications. Atropine 0.5-1.0 mg may be given IV if rate falls.

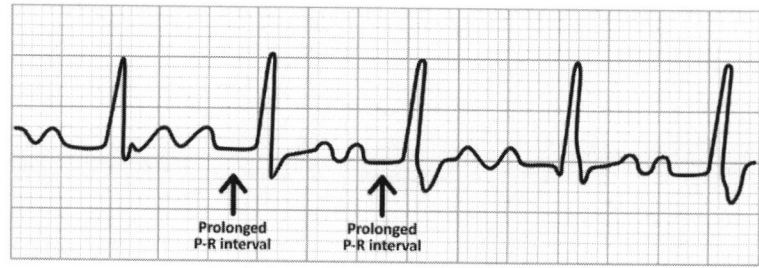

SECOND-DEGREE AV BLOCK

Second-degree AV block occurs when some of the atrial beats are blocked. Second-degree AV block is further subdivided according to the patterns of block.

TYPE I

Mobitz type I block (Wenckebach) occurs when each atrial impulse in a group of beats is conducted at a lengthened interval until one fails to conduct (the PR interval progressively increases), so there are more P waves than QRS complexes, but the QRS complex is usually of normal shape and duration. The sinus node functions at a regular rate, so the P-P interval is regular, but the R-R interval usually shortens with each impulse. The P:QRS ratio varies, such as 3:2, 4:3, 5:4. This type of block by itself usually does not cause significant morbidity unless associated with an inferior wall myocardial infarction.

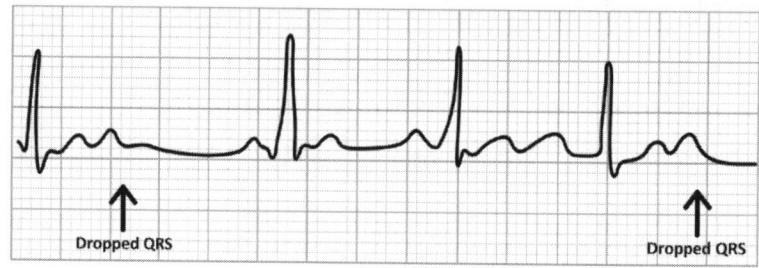

TYPE II

In Mobitz type II, only some of the atrial impulses are conducted unpredictably through the AV node to the ventricles, and the block always occurs below the AV node in the bundle of His, the bundle branches, or the Purkinje fibers. The PR intervals are the same if impulses are conducted, and the QRS complex is usually widened. The P:QRS ratio varies 2:1, 3:1, and 4:1. Type II block is more dangerous than Type I because it may progress to complete AV block and may produce Stokes-Adams syncope. Additionally, if the block is at the Purkinje fibers, there is no escape impulse. Usually, a transcutaneous cardiac pacemaker and defibrillator should be at the patient's bedside. **Symptoms** may include chest pain if the heart block is precipitated by myocarditis or myocardial ischemia.

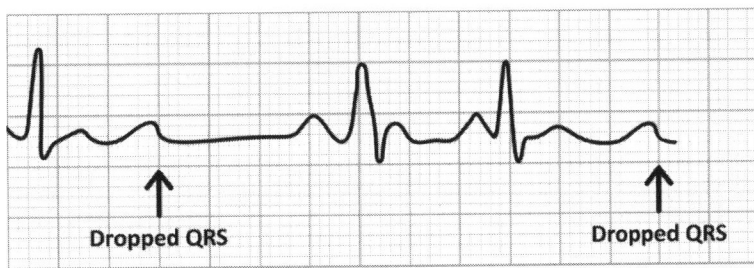

THIRD-DEGREE

With third-degree AV block, there are more P waves than QRS complexes, with no clear relationship between them. The atrial rate is 2-3 times the pulse rate, so the PR interval is irregular. If the SA node malfunctions, the AV node fires at a lower rate, and if the AV node malfunctions, the pacemaker site in the ventricles takes over at a bradycardic rate; thus, with complete AV block, the heart still contracts, but often ineffectually. With this type of block, the atrial P (sinus rhythm or atrial fibrillation) and the ventricular QRS (ventricular escape rhythm) are stimulated by different impulses, so there is AV dissociation.

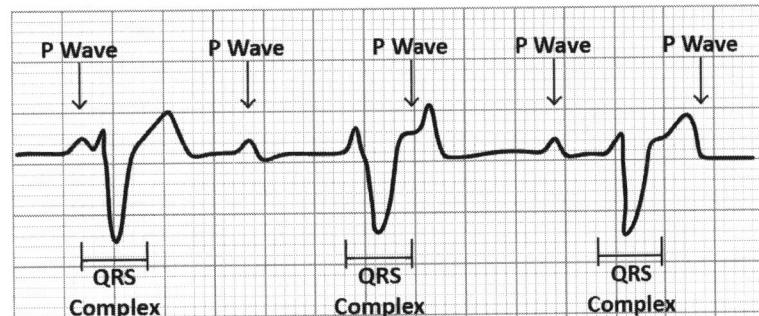

The heart may compensate at rest but can't keep pace with exertion. The resultant bradycardia may cause congestive heart failure, fainting, or even sudden death, and usually conduction abnormalities slowly worsen. **Symptoms** include dyspnea, chest pain, and hypotension, which are treated with IV atropine. Transcutaneous pacing may be needed. Complete persistent AV block normally requires implanted pacemakers, usually dual chamber.

> **Review Video: AV Heart Blocks**
> Visit mometrix.com/academy and enter code: 487004

BUNDLE BRANCH BLOCKS

A **right bundle branch block (RBBB)** occurs when conduction is blocked in the right bundle branch that carries impulses from the Bundle of His to the right ventricle. The impulse travels through the left ventricle instead, and then reaches the right ventricle, but this causes a slight delay in contraction of the right ventricle. A RBBB is characterized by normal P waves (as the right atrium still contracts appropriately), but the QRS complex is widened and notched (referred to as an "RSR pattern" that resembles the letter "M") in lead V1, which is a reflection of the asynchronous ventricular contraction. The PR interval is normal or prolonged, and the QRS interval is > 0.12 seconds. P:QRS ratio remains 1:1 with regular rhythms.

A **left bundle branch block (LBBB)** occurs when there is a delay in conduction between the left atrium and left ventricle. It is also characterized by normal or inverted P waves, but the QRS complex may be widened with a deep S wave and an interval of >0.12 seconds (in lead V1) that resembles a "W." The PR interval may be normal or prolonged. The P:QRS ratio is 1:1 and the rhythm is regular.

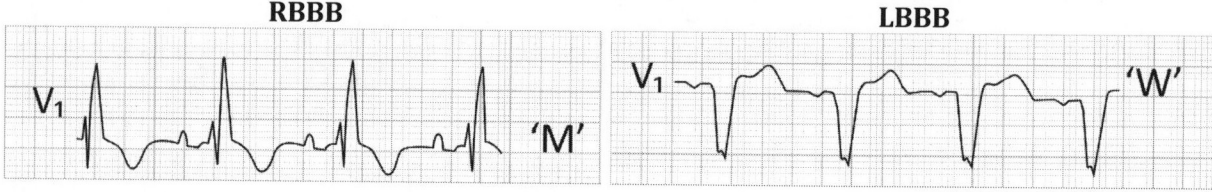

Heart Failure

Heart failure (formerly congestive heart failure) is a cardiac disease that includes disorders of contractions (systolic dysfunction) or filling (diastolic dysfunction) or both and may include pulmonary, peripheral, or systemic edema. The most common causes are coronary artery disease, systemic or pulmonary hypertension, cardiomyopathy, and valvular disorders. The incidence of chronic heart failure correlates with age. The 2 main types of HF are systolic and diastolic. HF is classified according to symptoms and prognosis:

- **Class I**: The patient is essentially asymptomatic during normal activities with no pulmonary congestion or peripheral hypotension. There is no restriction on activities, and prognosis is good.
- **Class II**: Symptoms appear with physical exertion but are usually absent at rest, resulting in some limitations of activities of daily living (ADLs). Slight pulmonary edema may be evident by basilar rales. Prognosis is good.
- **Class III**: Obvious limitations of ADLs and discomfort on any exertion. Prognosis is fair.
- **Class IV**: Symptoms at rest. Prognosis is poor.

Treatment may include:

- Careful monitoring of **fluid balance** and **weight** to determine changes in fluid retention
- **Low sodium diet**
- **Restriction of activity**
- **Medications** may include diuretics, vasodilators, or ACE inhibitors to decrease the heart's workload, digoxin may be given to increase contractibility
- **Anticoagulant therapy** if distended atria, enlarged ventricles, or atrial fibrillation to decrease the danger of thromboembolic

> **Review Video: Congestive Heart Failure**
> Visit mometrix.com/academy and enter code: 924118

Systolic Heart Failure

Systolic heart failure is the typical "left-sided" failure and reduces the amount of blood ejected from the ventricles during contraction (decreased ejection fraction). This stimulates the SNS to produce catecholamines to support the myocardium, which eventually causes down regulation, the destruction of beta and adrenergic receptor sites, and ultimately further myocardial damage. Because of reduced perfusion, the R-A-A pathway (renin, angiotensin I&II, aldosterone) is initiated by the kidneys, causing sodium and fluid retention. The end result of these processes is increased preload and afterload, thus increased workload on the ventricles. They begin to lose contractibility and blood begins to pool inside, stretching the myocardium (ventricular remodeling). The heart compensates by thickening the muscle (hypertrophy) without an adequate increase in capillary blood supply, leading to ischemia.

Symptoms: Activity intolerance, dyspnea/orthopnea (sleeping in a recliner is a classic symptom), cough (frothy sputum), edema, heart sounds S3 and S4, hepatomegaly, JVD, LOC changes, and tachycardia.

Treatment includes:

- Medication
- **Surgery**: Heart transplant (if a candidate)
- **Lifestyle modification**: Low-sodium diet, supplemental oxygen, daily weights (report >3 lb/day or 5 lb/week weight gain to physician)

DIASTOLIC HEART FAILURE

Diastolic heart failure may be difficult to differentiate from systolic heart failure based on clinical symptoms, which are similar. With diastolic heart failure, the myocardium is unable to sufficiently relax to facilitate filling of the ventricles. This may be the end result of systolic heart failure as myocardial hypertrophy stiffens the muscles, and the causes are similar. Diastolic heart failure is more common in females >75. Typically, intra-cardiac pressures at rest are within normal range but increase markedly on exertion. Because the relaxation of the heart is delayed, the ventricles do not expand enough for the fill-volume, and the heart cannot increase stroke volume during exercise, so symptoms (dyspnea, fatigue, pulmonary edema) are often pronounced on exertion. Ejection fractions are usually >40-50% with increase in left ventricular end-diastolic pressure (LVEDP) and decrease in left ventricular end-diastolic volume (LVEDV).

The major goal with all types of heart failure is to prevent further damage and remodeling, prevent exacerbations, and improve the patient's long-term prognosis.

ACUTE HEART FAILURE

Acute decompensated heart failure occurs when the body cannot compensate for the heart's inability to provide adequate perfusion. Cardiac output is no longer sufficient to meet the metabolic demands of the body. Acute heart failure occurs suddenly and can be precipitated by dysrhythmias, illness, noncompliance with medications, acute ischemia, fluid overload or hypertensive crisis. Acute heart failure is most commonly related to left ventricular systolic or diastolic dysfunction. It requires immediate treatment to restore adequate perfusion and is often life-threatening.

Signs and symptoms: Dyspnea, cough, edema, ascites and elevated jugular venous pressure, fatigue, cool extremities, hypotension and altered mental status

Diagnostic testing: Chest x-ray, electrocardiogram, physical exam; labs—basic metabolic panel, BUN, creatinine, and B-natriuretic peptide (BNP)

Treatment: Rapid assessment and stabilization of the patient. The physical assessment should include a thorough evaluation of the patient's respiratory status and supplemental oxygen and potentially ventilator support may be necessary. Medications: Diuretics to decrease fluid volume; vasodilators to decrease pulmonary congestion. Cardiac monitoring, urine output monitoring, sodium restriction, and venous thromboembolism prophylaxis may also be utilized.

HYPERTENSIVE CRISES

Hypertensive crises are marked elevations in blood pressure that can cause severe organ damage if left untreated. Hypertensive crises may be caused by endocrine/renal disorders (pheochromocytoma), dissection of an aortic aneurysm, pulmonary edema, subarachnoid hemorrhage, stroke, eclampsia, and medication noncompliance. There are two **classifications**:

- **Hypertensive emergency** occurs when acute hypertension, usually >220 systolic and 120 mmHg diastolic, must be treated immediately to lower blood pressure in order to prevent damage to vital organs.
- **Hypertensive urgency** occurs when acute hypertension must be treated within a few hours but the vital organs are not in immediate danger. Blood pressure is lowered more slowly to avoid hypotension, ischemia of vital organs, or failure of autoregulation.
  - 1/3 reduction in 6 hours
  - 1/3 reduction in next 24 hours
  - 1/3 reduction over days 2-4

Symptoms: Basilar HA, blurred vision, chest pain, N/V, SOB, seizures, ruddy pallor, and anxiety

Diagnostics: ECG, Chest x-ray, CBC, BMP, Urinalysis (+ blood and casts)

Treatment includes:

- Medications: Vasodilators (Cardene, Nitro, etc.) and diuretics
- Nursing Interventions: Raise HOB to 90°, supplemental O_2, frequent neuro checks, teach concerning medication compliance

ENDOCARDITIS

Endocarditis is an infection of the lining of the heart that covers the heart valves and contains Purkinje fibers, known as the endocardium. Risk factors include being over 60 years of age, being male, IV drug use, and dental infections. Staphylococcal aureus is the most common cause of infective endocarditis. Etiology includes subacute bacterial endocarditis (often related to dental procedures), prosthetic valvular endocarditis (following valve replacement), and right sided endocarditis (often related to catheter infections and IV drug use). Organisms enter the bloodstream from portals of entry (surgery, catheterization, IV drug abuse) and migrate to the heart, growing on the endothelial tissue and forming vegetations (verrucae), collagen deposits, and platelet thrombi. With endocarditis, the valves frequently become deformed, but the pathogenic agents may also invade other tissues, such as the chordae tendineae. The lesions may invade adjacent tissue and break off, becoming emboli. The mitral valve is the most common valve affected, followed by aortic, tricuspid, and the pulmonary valve being the least often affected. Positive blood cultures, widened pulse pressures, ECG, murmurs, and vegetations seen on a transesophageal echocardiogram are used to make the diagnosis. After diagnosis is made, antibiotics are used for treatment, and when unsuccessful or when heart failure is present, valve repair may be warranted. Serious complications from endocarditis include emboli, sepsis, and heart failure. Untreated endocarditis is fatal.

DIAGNOSIS AND TREATMENT

Diagnosis of endocarditis is made on the basis of clinical presentation and **diagnostic procedures** that may include:

- **Blood cultures** should be done with 3 sets for both aerobic and anaerobic bacteria. Diagnosis is definitive if 2 cultures are positive, but a negative culture does not preclude bacterial endocarditis.
- **Echocardiogram** may identify vegetation on valves or increasing heart failure
- **ECG** may demonstrate prolonged PR interval
- **Anemia** (normochromic, normocytic)
- Elevated **white blood cell count**
- Elevated **erythrocyte sedimentation rate** (ESR) and **C-reactive protein** (CRP)

Treatment includes general management of symptoms and the following:

- **Antimicrobials** specific to the pathogenic organism, usually administered IV for 4 to 6 weeks
- **Surgical replacement** of aortic and/or mitral valves may be necessary (in 30% to 40% of cases) if there is no response to treatment and/or after infection is controlled if there are severe symptoms related to valve damage

CLINICAL SYMPTOMS

Clinical symptoms of endocarditis usually relate to the response to infection, the underlying heart disease, emboli, or immunological response. Typical **symptoms** include:

- Slow onset with unexplained low-grade and often intermittent **fever**
- **Anorexia** and weight loss, difficulty feeding
- General **lassitude** and malaise
- **Splenomegaly** present in 60% of patients; **hepatomegaly** may also be present
- **Anemia** is present in almost all patients
- Sudden **aortic valve insufficiency** or mitral valve insufficiency
- **Cyanosis** with clubbing of fingers
- **Embolism** of other body organs (brain, liver, bones)
- **Congestive heart failure**
- **Dysrhythmias**
- New or change in **heart murmur**
- **Immunological responses**
- **Janeway lesions**: painless areas of hemorrhage on palms of hands and soles of feet
- **Splinter hemorrhages**: thin, brown-black lines on nails of fingers and toes
- **Petechiae**: pinpoint-sized hemorrhages on oral mucous membranes, as well as hands and trunk
- **Roth spots**: retinal hemorrhagic lesions caused by emboli on nerve fibers
- **Glomerulonephritis**: microscopic hematuria

MYOCARDITIS

Myocarditis is inflammation of the cardiac myocardium (muscle tissue), usually triggered by a viral infection, such as the influenza virus, Coxsackie virus, and HIV. Myocarditis can also be caused by bacteria, fungi, or parasites, or an allergic response to medications. In some cases, it is also a complication of endocarditis. It may also be triggered by chemotherapy drugs and some antibiotics.

Myocarditis can result in dilation of the heart, development of thrombi on the heart walls (known as mural thrombi), and infiltration of blood cells around the coronary vessels and between muscle fibers, causing further degeneration of the muscle tissue. The heart may become enlarged and weak, as the ability to pump blood is impaired, leading to congestive heart failure. Symptoms depend upon the extent of damage but may include fatigue, dyspnea, pressure and discomfort in chest or epigastric area, and palpitations.

DIAGNOSIS AND TREATMENT

Diagnosis of myocarditis depends upon the clinical picture, as there is no test specific for myocarditis, although a number of tests may be done to verify the **clinical diagnosis**:

- **Chest radiograph** may indicate cardiomegaly or pulmonary edema.
- **ECG** may show nonspecific changes.
- **Echocardiogram** may indicate cardiomegaly and demonstrate defects in functioning.
- **Cardiac catheterization** and **cardiac biopsy** will yield confirmation in 65% of cases, but not all of the heart muscle may be affected, so a negative finding does not rule out myocarditis.
- **Viral cultures** of nasopharynx and rectal may help to identify organism.
- **Viral titers** may increase as disease progresses.
- **Polymerase chain reaction** (PCR) of biopsy specimen may be most effective for diagnosis.

Treatment:

- As indicated for underlying cause (such as antibiotics)
- Restriction of activities
- Careful **monitoring** for heart failure and medical treatment as indicated (e.g., diuretics, digoxin)
- **Oxygen** as needed to maintain normal oxygen saturation
- **IV gamma globulin** for acute stage

ACUTE PERICARDITIS

Pericarditis is inflammation of the pericardial sac with or without increased pericardial fluid. It may be an isolated process or the effect of an underlying disease. If the underlying cause is autoimmune or related to malignancy of some sort, the patient usually presents with symptoms that relate to that disorder. However, most cases are related to a viral etiology, and therefore usually present with flu-like symptoms. Patients that have idiopathic pericarditis or viral pericarditis have a good prognosis with medication alone.

Signs/Symptoms: Sharp chest pain, worsened with inspiration and relieved by leaning forward or sitting up (most common symptom; "Mohammad's Sign"), pericardial effusion, respiratory distress, auscultated friction rub, ST elevation/PR depression (progresses to flattened T, inverted T, then return to normal); risk of pericardial effusion.

Diagnosis: Echocardiogram, ECG, pericardiocentesis or pericardial biopsy, cardiac enzymes (may be mildly elevated), WBC/ESR/CRP all elevated.

Treatment includes:

- **Medications**: NSAIDs for pain/inflammation, Colchicine 0.5 mg twice a day for six months is often prescribed in adjunct to NSAID therapy, as it decreases the incidence of recurrence
- **Surgery**: Pericardiectomy only in extreme cases

ACUTE CARDIAC-RELATED PULMONARY EDEMA

Acute cardiac-related pulmonary edema occurs when heart failure results in fluid overload, leading to third-spacing of fluid into the interstitial spaces of the lungs. Pulmonary edema may result from MI, chronic HF, volume overload, ischemia, or mitral stenosis.

Symptoms include severe dyspnea, cough with blood-tinged frothy sputum, wheezing/rales/crackles on auscultation, cyanosis, and diaphoresis.

Diagnosis: Auscultation, chest x-ray, and echocardiogram.

Treatment includes:

- Sitting position with 100% oxygen by mask to achieve PO_2 >60%
- Non-invasive pressure support ventilation (BiPAP) or endotracheal intubation and mechanical ventilation
- Morphine sulfate 2-8 mg (IV for severe cases), repeated every 2-4 hours as needed—decreases pre-load and anxiety
- IV diuretics (furosemide ≥40 mg or bumetanide ≥1 mg) to provide venous dilation and diuresis
- Nitrates as a bolus with an infusion—decreases pre-load
- Inhaled β-adrenergic agonists or aminophylline for bronchospasm
- Digoxin IV for tachycardia
- ACE inhibitors, nitroprusside to reduce afterload

VALVULAR DISORDERS

MITRAL STENOSIS

Mitral stenosis is a narrowing of the mitral valve that allows blood to flow from the left atrium to the left ventricle. Pressure in the left atrium increases to overcome resistance, resulting in enlargement of the left atrium and increased pressure in the pulmonary veins and capillaries of the lung (pulmonary hypertension). Mitral stenosis can be caused by infective endocarditis, calcifications, or tumors in the left atrium.

Signs/Symptoms: Exertional dyspnea, orthopnea/nocturnal dyspnea, right-sided heart failure, loud S_1 and S_2, and mid-diastolic murmur.

Diagnosis: Cardiac catheterization, chest x-ray, echocardiogram, ECG.

Treatment includes:

- **Medications**: Antiarrhythmic, anticoagulant, and antihypertensive medications
- **Surgical**: Open/closed commissurotomy, balloon valvuloplasty, and mitral valve replacement

MITRAL VALVE INSUFFICIENCY

Mitral valve insufficiency occurs when the mitral valve fails to close completely so that there is backflow into the left atrium from the left ventricle during systole, decreasing cardiac output. It may occur with mitral stenosis or independently. Mitral valve insufficiency can result from damage caused by rheumatic fever, myxomatous degeneration, infective endocarditis, collagen vascular disease (Marfan's syndrome), or cardiomyopathy/left heart failure. There are **three phases** of the disease:

- **Acute**: May occur with rupture of a chordae tendineae or papillary muscle causing sudden left ventricular flooding and overload.
- **Chronic compensated**: Enlargement of the left atrium to decrease filling pressure, and hypertrophy of the left ventricle.
- **Chronic decompensated**: Left ventricle fails to compensate for the volume overload; decreased stroke volume and increased cardiac output.

Symptoms: Orthopnea/dyspnea, split $S_2/S_3/S_4$ heart sounds, systolic murmur, palpitations, right-sided heart failure, fatigue, angina (rare).

Diagnosis: Cardiac catheterization, chest x-ray, echocardiogram, ECG.

Treatment includes:

- **Medications**: Antiarrhythmic, anticoagulant, and antihypertensive medications.
- **Surgical**: Annuloplasty or valvuloplasty, and mitral valve replacement.

AORTIC STENOSIS

Aortic stenosis is a stricture (narrowing) of the aortic valve that controls the flow of blood from the left ventricle. This causes the left ventricular wall to thicken as it increases pressure to overcome the valvular resistance, increasing afterload and increasing the need for blood supply from the coronary arteries. This condition may result from a birth defect or childhood rheumatic fever, and tends to worsen over the years as the heart grows.

Symptoms: Angina, exercise intolerance, dyspnea, split S_1 and S_2, systolic murmur at base of carotids, hypotension on exertion, syncope, left-sided heart failure; sudden death can occur.

Diagnosis: Cardiac catheterization, chest x-ray, echocardiogram, ECG.

Treatment includes:

- **Medications**: Antiarrhythmic, anticoagulant, and antihypertensive medications
- **Surgical**: Balloon valvuloplasty, and aortic valve replacement

PULMONIC STENOSIS

Pulmonic stenosis is a stricture of the pulmonary blood that controls the flow of blood from the right ventricle to the lungs, resulting in right ventricular hypertrophy as the pressure increases in the right ventricle and decreased pulmonary blood flow. The condition may be asymptomatic or symptoms may not be evident until adulthood, depending upon the severity of the defect. Pulmonic stenosis may be associated with a number of other heart defects.

Symptoms: May be asymptomatic; dyspnea on exertion, systolic heart murmur, right-sided heart failure.

Diagnosis: Cardiac catheterization, chest x-ray, echocardiogram, ECG.

Treatment includes:

- **Medications**: Antiarrhythmic, anticoagulant, and antihypertensive medications
- **Surgical**: Balloon valvuloplasty, valvotomy, valvectomy with or without transannular patch, and pulmonary valve replacement

37

Vascular Conditions

PERIPHERAL ARTERIAL AND VENOUS INSUFFICIENCY

Characteristics of peripheral arterial and venous insufficiency are listed below:

- **Arterial insufficiency**
  - **Pain**: Ranging from intermittent claudication to severe and constant shooting pain
  - **Pulses**: Weak or absent
  - **Skin**: Rubor on dependency, but pallor of foot on elevation; pale, shiny, and cool skin with loss of hair on toes and foot; nails thick and ridged
  - **Ulcers**: Painful, deep, circular, often necrotic ulcers on toe tips, toe webs, heels, or other pressure areas
  - **Edema**: Minimal
- **Venous insufficiency**
  - **Pain**: Aching/cramping
  - **Pulses**: Strong/present
  - **Skin**: Brownish discoloration around ankles and anterior tibial area
  - **Ulcers**: Varying degrees of pain in superficial, irregular ulcers on medial or lateral malleolus and sometimes the anterior tibial area
  - **Edema**: Moderate to severe

ACUTE PERIPHERAL VASCULAR INSUFFICIENCY

Acute peripheral arterial insufficiency can occur when sudden occlusion of a blood vessel causes tissue ischemia, ultimately leading to cellular death and necrosis. This can occur as a result of traumatic injury or non-traumatic events such as arterial thrombus or embolism, vasospasm, or severe swelling (compartment syndrome). Risk factors for acute peripheral arterial insufficiency include age, tobacco use, diabetes mellitus, hyperlipidemia, and hypertension.

- **Signs and symptoms**: Classic 6 P's: Pain (extreme, unrelieved by narcotics), pallor, pulselessness, poikilothermia (the inability to regulate body temperature; extremity is room temperature), paresthesias, and paralysis (late).
- **Diagnosis**: Ultrasound, angiography, and physical exam; labs—coagulation studies, CBC, BMP, creatinine phosphokinase
- **Treatment**: Re-establishment of blood flow to the affected area
- **Arterial thrombus or embolism**: Mechanical thrombolysis may be performed to remove the clot occluding the vessel.
  - **Trauma**: Surgical repair of the severed/injured vessels. Fasciotomy may be performed in the event of compartment syndrome to relieve pressure.
  - **Other treatment options**: Hyperbaric oxygen therapy, anti-platelet therapy for the prevention of arterial thrombosis and anti-coagulant therapy for the prevention of venous thrombosis

ACUTE VENOUS THROMBOEMBOLISM

Acute venous thromboembolism (VTE) is a condition that includes both deep vein thrombosis (DVT) and pulmonary emboli (PE). VTE may be precipitated by invasive procedures, lack of mobility, and inflammation, so it is a common complication in critical care units. **Virchow's triad** comprises common risk factors: blood stasis, injury to endothelium, and hypercoagulability. Some patients may be initially asymptomatic, but **symptoms** may include:

- Aching or throbbing pain
- Positive Homan's sign (pain in calf when foot is dorsiflexed)
- Unilateral erythema and edema
- Dilation of vessels
- Cyanosis

Diagnosis: ultrasound and/or D-dimer test, which tests the serum for cross-linked fibrin derivatives. A CT scan, pulmonary angiogram, and ventilation-perfusion lung scan may be used to diagnose pulmonary emboli.

Treatment includes:

- Medications: IV heparin, tPA, or other anticoagulation; analgesia for pain
- Surgical: May have to surgically remove clot if large
- Bed rest, elevation of affected limb; stockings on ambulation

Prevention: Use of sequential compression devices (SCDs) or foot pumps, routine anticoagulant use for those at highest risk (Heparin SQ), early and frequent ambulation

> **Review Video: DVT Prevention and Treatment**
> Visit mometrix.com/academy and enter code: 234086

AORTIC ANEURYSMS

TYPES

A **dissecting aortic aneurysm** occurs when the wall of the aorta is torn and blood flows between the layers of the wall, dilating and weakening it until it risks rupture (which has a 90% mortality). Aortic aneurysms are more than twice as common in males as females, but females have a higher mortality rate, possibly due to increased age at diagnosis.

Abdominal aortic aneurysms (AAA) are usually related to atherosclerosis, but may also result from Marfan syndrome, Ehlers-Danlos disease, and connective tissue disorders. Rupture usually does not allow time for emergent repair, so identifying and correcting before rupture is essential. Different classification systems are used to describe the type and degree of dissection. Common classification:

- **DeBakey classification** uses anatomic location as the focal point:
  - Type I begins in the ascending aorta but may spread to include the aortic arch and the descending aorta (60%). This is also considered a proximal lesion or Stanford type A.
  - Type II is restricted to the ascending aorta (10-15%). This is also considered a proximal lesion or Stanford type A.
  - Type III is restricted to the descending aorta (25-30%). This is considered a distal lesion or Stanford type B.
- Types I and II are thoracic, and type III is abdominal.

39

DIAGNOSIS AND TREATMENT

Aortic aneurysms are often asymptomatic, but when symptomatic, patients present with substernal pain, back pain, dyspnea and/or stridor (from pressure on trachea), cough, distention of neck veins, palpable and pulsating abdominal mass, edema of neck and arms.

Diagnosis: x-ray, CT, MRI, Cardiac catheterization, TEE/transthoracic echocardiogram.

Treatment includes:

- **Anti-hypertensives** to reduce systolic BP, such as β-blockers (esmolol) or Alpha-β-blocker combinations (labetalol) to reduce force of blood as it leaves the ventricle to reduce pressure against the aortic wall. IV vasodilators (sodium nitroprusside) may also be needed.
- **Intubation and ventilation** may be required if the patient is hemodynamically unstable.
- **Analgesia/sedation** to control anxiety and pain.
- **Surgical repair**: Types I and II are usually repaired surgically because of the danger of rupture and cardiac tamponade. Type III (abdominal) is often followed medically and surgically only if the aneurysm is >5.5cm or rapidly expanding. There are two types of surgical repair:
    - **Open**: Patient is placed on cardiopulmonary bypass, and through an abdominal incision the damaged portion is removed, and a graft is sutured in place.
    - **Endovascular**: A stent graft is fed through the arteries to line the aorta and exclude the aneurysm.

Complications: Myocardial infarction, renal injury, and GI hemorrhage/ischemic bowel, which may occur up to years after surgery. Endo-leaks can occur with a stent graft, increasing risk of rupture.

AORTIC RUPTURE

Aortic rupture is a catastrophic breakage of the aorta, generally as the result of trauma or rupture of an aortic aneurysm. **Aortic rupture** (spontaneous) most commonly occurs in the abdominal aorta. The patient typically experiences a severe tearing pain and loses consciousness from hypovolemic shock as the blood pours out of the aorta. Tachycardia occurs and the patient may exhibit cyanosis. An ecchymotic area may appear in the flank area because of retroperitoneal pooling of blood. Diagnostic tests include ultrasound or CT. Survival depends on the size of the tear, the amount of blood loss, and the length of time until surgical repair. About 90% of patients die prior to surgery. An aortic occlusion balloon to stem bleeding may be placed temporarily in order to stabilize the patient. Surgical repair may be via an open procedure or endovascular therapy. Risk factors include male gender, older age, smoking, history of MI, family history of abdominal aortic aneurysm, peripheral arterial disease, and hypertension.

HYPERLIPIDEMIA
CAUSES AND IMPACT ON CARDIAC FUNCTION

Hyperlipidemia, particularly increased low-density lipoproteins (LDL), decreased high density lipoproteins (HDL), and increased triglycerides, are associated with increased risk of coronary heart disease, especially with other risk factors present, such as hypertension, diabetes mellitus, older age, male gender, and history of smoking. The causes of hyperlipidemia may include a number of additional factors, including genetic factors, high fat diet, obesity, and excessive intake of alcohol. Some other disorders, such renal disease and hypothyroidism, are also associated with hyperlipidemia. LDLs increase atherosclerosis by accumulating in plagues on the walls of vessels, leading to impaired circulation and risk of clot formation. HDLs, on the other hand, transport excess cholesterol to the liver so it can be broken down and excreted. Triglycerides are carried by chylomicron (which reflect fat intake after a meal) and very-low density lipoprotein (VLDL) (which increase when fasting and reflect carbohydrate intake). After VLDL releases triglycerides for energy, they eventually become LDL with small particles that increase risk of cardiovascular events. Both VLDL and chylomicrons increase inflammation of arterial endothelium.

LAB VALUES THAT INDICATE HYPERLIPIDEMIA

The NIH, NHLBI Report of the National Cholesterol Education Program Expert Panel on Detection, Evaluation, and Treatment of high Blood Cholesterol in Adults classifies total cholesterol, LDL, and HDL to help to determine the need for treatment. Classification includes:

LDL cholesterol	$< 100 =$ Optimal
	$100 - 129 =$ Near optimal
	$130 - 159 =$ Borderline high
	$160 - 189 =$ High
	$\geq 190 =$ Very high
Total cholesterol	$< 200 =$ Optimal
	$200 - 239 =$ Borderline high
	$\geq 240 =$ High
HDL cholesterol	$< 40 =$ Low
	$\geq 60 =$ High (optimal)
Triglycerides	$< 150 =$ Normal
	$150 - 199 =$ Borderline $-$ high
	$200 - 499 =$ High
	$\geq 500 =$ Very high

The optimal LDL goal for those with CHD or equivalent risk is < 100 mg/dL; 0-1 risk factors, <160 mg/dL; and more than 2 risk factors, <160 mg/dL. Those with coronary heart disease or equivalent risk factor have a risk of having major coronary events at the rate of >20% per 10 years.

THERAPEUTIC INTERVENTIONS

HMG-CoA REDUCTASE INHIBITORS (STATINS)

HMG-CoA reductase inhibitors, known as statins, inhibit an enzyme necessary for the production of cholesterol, reduce synthesis of cholesterol in the liver, and increase hepatic LDL receptors (which increase uptake and reduce circulating LDL). High intensity statins (statins administered at higher doses) reduce LDL by greater than 50% while moderate intensity statins (administered at lower doses) reduce LDL by 30-50% with lesser effects on increasing HDL and lowering triglycerides:

- Atorvastatin (Lipitor) 10-80 mg/day
- Fluvastatin (Lescol XL) 20-80 mg/day
- Lovastatin (Altoprev) 20-80 mg/day
- Pitavastatin (Livalo) 1-4 mg/day
- Rosuvastatin (Crestor)5-40 mg/day
- Simvastatin (Zocor) 20-40 mg/day

EZETIMIBE

Ezetimibe inhibits the absorption of dietary and biliary cholesterol through intestinal wall, reducing LDL by up to 20% or more (if used in combined therapy). Dosage is 10 mg daily.

BILE ACID BINDING RESINS

Bile acid binding resins bind bile acids in the intestines, decreasing absorption and causing the liver to use hepatic cholesterol to increase production of bile acids to compensate, lowering circulating LDL. They have no effect on triglycerides:

- Cholestyramine (Questran) 8-26 g divided doses
- Colesevelam (Welchol) 3750 mg once daily or in divided doses
- Colestipol (Colestid) 5-30 g divided doses

FIBRIC ACID DERIVATIVES

Fibric acid derivatives reduce plasma triglycerides by up to 40%, increase HDL by up to 20%, and reduce LDL by up to 20%. They are used primarily to treat elevated triglycerides:

- Fenofibrate (Tricor, Antara, Lipofen, Fenoglide) 48-145 mg q day (dosages may vary slightly from one brand to another).
- Gemfibrozil (Lopid) 600mg/day to 600 mg BID.

DIET

Low fat diet limits saturated and trans fats and encourage fruits, vegetables, lean protein meat, nuts, and whole grains with limited refined carbohydrates and increased fiber. Effects on cholesterol levels vary but reduce LDL by up to 10% for most patients.

VASCULAR INTERVENTION LEADINGS TO COMPLICATIONS

RETROPERITONEAL BLEEDING

Retroperitoneal bleeding may occur as a complication of femoral artery catheterization (such as for PCI procedures) when the artery is perforated or dissected. A large hematoma forms and dissects the artery with bleeding into the retroperitoneum, a life-threatening complication. Factors that increase the risk of perforation include large catheter size, multiple attempts at insertion, long dwell time, inadequate vascular closure, and accidental perforation. Risk of severe hemorrhage is increased with the use of periprocedural anticoagulation and antiplatelet agents. Patients of older age and large size/body weight as well as those with preexisting coagulopathy, hypertension, and renal disease also have increased risk. With bleeding, patients may complain of abdominal, back, or groin pain or swelling, and some may exhibit unexplained hypotension and bradycardia or tachycardia. Diagnosis is confirmed by symptoms and CT. Treatment includes blood transfusions and surgical repair.

PSEUDOANEURYSMS

Pseudoaneurysm (AKA false aneurysm), which is injury to the inner layers of the arterial wall allowing blood to collect and balloon out between the two outer layers of the arterial wall, results in a thin-walled cavity that is prone to rupture. If all 3 layers of the artery are disrupted, the blood may be contained by surrounding tissue. A pseudoaneurysm may occur with injury to the arterial wall during PCI procedures, especially with femoral catheterization. Blood may leak and pool at the insertion site. Contributing factors include periprocedural anticoagulation, inadequate compression of the insertion site after removal of the catheter, hypertension, and arterial calcifications. Patients may complain of pain about insertion site with a pulsatile mass evident on examination and with a systolic bruit. Diagnosis is per Doppler ultrasound or color flow imaging. Treatment includes close monitoring as small pseudoaneurysms may heal spontaneously, ultrasound-guided compression, ultrasound-guided thrombin injection, or surgical repair.

Non-Cardiovascular Conditions

Respiratory

ACUTE PULMONARY EMBOLISM

Acute pulmonary embolism occurs when a pulmonary artery or arteriole is blocked, cutting off blood supply to the pulmonary vessels and subsequent oxygenation of the blood. While most pulmonary emboli are from thrombus formation, they can also be caused by air, fat, or septic embolus (from bacterial invasion of a thrombus). Common originating sites for thrombus formation are the deep veins in the legs, the pelvic veins, and the right atrium. Causes include stasis related to damage to endothelial wall and changes in blood coagulation factors. Atrial fibrillation poses a serious risk because blood pools in the right atrium, forming clots that travel directly through the right ventricle to the lungs. The obstruction of the artery/arteriole causes an increase in alveolar dead space in which there is ventilation but impairment of gas exchange because of the ventilation/perfusion mismatching or intrapulmonary shunting. This results in hypoxia, hypercapnia, and the release of mediators that cause bronchoconstriction. If more than 50% of the vascular bed becomes excluded, pulmonary hypertension occurs.

SYMPTOMS AND DIAGNOSIS

Clinical manifestations of acute pulmonary embolism (PE) vary according to the size of the embolus and the area of occlusion.

Symptoms include:

- Dyspnea with tachypnea
- Cyanosis; may turn grey or blue from nipple line up (massive PE)
- Anxiety and restlessness, feeling of doom
- Chest pain, tachycardia, may progress to arrhythmias (PEA)
- Fever
- Rales
- Cough (sometimes with hemoptysis)
- Hemodynamic instability

Diagnostic tests are as follows:

- ABG analysis may show hypoxemia (decreased PaO_2), hypocarbia (decreased $PaCO_2$) and respiratory alkalosis (increased pH).
- D-dimer will show elevation with PE but is not definitively diagnostic without a CT scan.
- ECG may show sinus tachycardia or other abnormalities.
- Echocardiogram can show emboli in the central arteries and can assess the hemodynamic status of the right side of the heart.
- Spiral CT may provide definitive diagnosis.
- V/Q scintigraphy can confirm diagnosis.
- Pulmonary angiograms also can confirm diagnosis.

MEDICAL MANAGEMENT

Medical management of pulmonary embolism starts with preventive measures for those at risk, including leg exercises, elastic compression stockings, and anticoagulation therapy. Most

43

pulmonary emboli present as medical emergencies, so the immediate task is to stabilize the patient. **Medical management** may include:

- **Oxygen** to relieve hypoxemia
- **Intravenous infusions:** Dobutamine (Dobutrex®) or dopamine (Intropin®) to relieve hypotension
- **Cardiac monitoring** for dysrhythmias and issues due to right sided heart failure
- **Medications** as indicated: digitalis glycosides, diuretic, and antiarrhythmics
- Intubation and mechanical ventilation may be required
- **Analgesics** (such as morphine sulfate) or sedation to relieve anxiety
- **Anticoagulants** to prevent recurrence (although it will not dissolve clots already present), including heparin and warfarin (Coumadin®)
- **Placement of percutaneous venous filter** (Greenfield) in the inferior vena cava to prevent further emboli from entering the lungs, if anticoagulation therapy is contraindicated
- **Thrombolytic therapy,** recombinant tissue-type plasminogen activator (rt-PA) or streptokinase, for those severely compromised, but these treatments have limited success and pose the danger of bleeding

ACUTE LUNG INJURY AND ACUTE RESPIRATORY DISTRESS SYNDROME

Acute lung injury (ALI) comprises a syndrome of respiratory distress culminating in acute respiratory distress syndrome (ARDS). ARDS is a dangerous, potentially fatal respiratory condition, always caused by an illness or injury to the lungs. Lung injury causes fluid to leak into the spaces between the alveoli and capillaries, increasing pressure on the alveoli, causing them to collapse. With increased fluid accumulation in the lungs, the ability of the lungs to move oxygen into the blood is decreased, resulting in hypoxemia. Lung injury also causes a release of cytokines, a type of inflammatory protein, which then brings neutrophils to the lung. These proteins and cells leak into nearby blood vessels and cause inflammation throughout the body. This immune response, in combination with low levels of blood oxygen, can lead to organ failure. Symptoms are characterized by respiratory distress within 72 hours of surgery or a serious injury to a person with otherwise normal lungs and no cardiac disorder. Untreated, the condition results in respiratory failure, MODS, and a mortality rate of 5-30%.

Symptoms include:

- Refractory hypoxemia (hypoxemia not responding to increasing levels of oxygen)
- Crackling rales/wheezing in lungs
- Decrease in pulmonary compliance which results in increased tachypnea with expiratory grunting
- Cyanosis/skin mottling
- Hypotension and tachycardia
- Symptoms associated with volume overload are missing (3rd heart sound or JVD)
- Respiratory alkalosis initially but, as the disease progresses, replaced with hypercarbia and respiratory acidosis
- Normal x-ray initially but then diffuse infiltrates in both lungs, while the heart and vessels appear normal

MANAGEMENT

The management of acute respiratory distress syndrome (ARDS) involves providing adequate gas exchange and preventing further damage to the lung from forced ventilation.

Treatment includes:

- Mechanical ventilation to maintain oxygenation and ventilation
- Corticosteroids (may increase mortality rates in some patient populations, though this is the most commonly given treatment), nitrous oxide, inhaled surfactant, and anti-inflammatory medications
- Treatment of the underlying condition is the only proven treatment, especially identifying and treating an infection with appropriate antibiotics, as sepsis is most common etiology for ARDS, but prophylactic antibiotics are not indicated.
- Conservative fluid management is indicated to reduce days on the ventilator, but does not reduce overall mortality.

Pharmacologic preventive care: Enoxaparin 40 mg subcutaneously QD, sucralfate 1 g NGT four times daily or omeprazole 40 mg IV QD, and enteral nutrition support within 24 hours of ICU admission or intubation.

VENTILATION MANAGEMENT

Ventilation management in ARDS consists of the following:

- O_2 therapy by nasal prongs, cannula, or mask may be sufficient in very mild cases to maintain oxygen saturation above 90%. Oxygen should be administered at 100% because of the mismatch between ventilation (V) and perfusion (Q), which can result in hypoxia on position change.
- ARDS oxygenation goal is PaO_2 55-80 mmHg or SpO_2 88-95%.
- Endotracheal intubation may be needed if SpO_2 falls or CO_2 levels rise.
- The ARDS Network recommends low tidal volumes (6 mL/kg) and higher PEEP (12 cmH$_2$O or more).
- The low tidal volume ventilation described above is referred to as lung protective ventilation, and it has been shown to reduce mortality in patients with ARDS.
- Placing patients with severe ARDS in prone position for 18-24 hours per day with chest and pelvis supported and abdomen unsupported allows the diaphragm to move posteriorly, increasing functional residual capacity (FRC) in many patients.

ACUTE RESPIRATORY FAILURE

CARDINAL SIGNS

The cardinal signs of respiratory failure include:

- Tachypnea
- Tachycardia
- Anxiety and restlessness
- Diaphoresis

Symptoms may vary according to the cause. An obstruction may cause more obvious respiratory symptoms than other disorders.

- Early signs may include changes in the depth and pattern of respirations with flaring nares, sternal retractions, expiratory grunting, wheezing, and extended expiration as the body tries to compensate for hypoxemia and increasing levels of carbon dioxide.
- Cyanosis may be evident.
- Central nervous depression, with alterations in consciousness occurs with decreased perfusion to the brain.
- As the hypoxemia worsens, cardiac arrhythmias, including bradycardia, may occur with either hypotension or hypertension.
- Dyspnea becomes more pronounced with depressed respirations.
- Eventually stupor, coma, and death can occur if the condition is not reversed.

HYPOXEMIC AND HYPERCAPNIC RESPIRATORY FAILURE

Hypoxemic respiratory failure occurs suddenly when gaseous exchange of oxygen for carbon dioxide cannot keep up with demand for oxygen or production of carbon dioxide:

- PaO_2 <60 mmHg
- $PaCO_2$ >40 mmHg
- Arterial pH <7.35

Hypoxemic respiratory failure can be the result of low inhaled oxygen, as at high elevations or with smoke inhalation. The following ventilatory mechanisms may be involved:

- Alveolar hypotension
- Ventilation-perfusion mismatch (the most common cause)
- Intrapulmonary shunts
- Diffusion impairment

Hypercapnic respiratory failure results from an increase in $PaCO_2$ >45-50 mmHg associated with respiratory acidosis and may include:

- Reduction in minute ventilation, total volume of gas ventilated in one minute (often related to neurological, muscle, or chest wall disorders, drug overdoses, or obstruction of upper airway)
- Increased dead space with wasted ventilation (related to lung disease or disorders of chest wall, such as scoliosis)
- Increased production of CO_2 (usually related to infection, burns, or other causes of hypermetabolism)
- Oxygen saturation normal or below normal

UNDERLYING CAUSES

There are a number of underlying causes for respiratory failure:

- **Airway obstruction:** Obstruction may result from an inhaled object or from an underlying disease process, such as cystic fibrosis, asthma, pulmonary edema, or infection.
- **Inadequate respirations:** This is a common cause among adults, especially related to obesity and sleep apnea. It may also be induced by an overdose of sedation medications such as opioids.
- **Neuromuscular disorders:** Those disorders that interfere with the neuromuscular functioning of the lungs or the chest wall, such as muscular dystrophy or spinal cord injuries can prevent adequate ventilation.
- **Pulmonary abnormalities:** Those abnormalities of the lung tissue, found in pulmonary fibrosis, burns, ARDS, and reactions to drugs, can lead to failure.
- **Chest wall abnormalities:** Disorders that impact lung parenchyma, such as severe scoliosis or chest wounds can interfere with lung functioning.

Nursing interventions to help prevent respiratory issues:

- Turn, position, and ambulate the patient.
- Have the patient cough and breathe deeply.
- Use vibration and percussion treatments.
- Hydrate the patient to help hydrate the airway secretions, and incentive spirometry.

MANAGEMENT

Respiratory failure must be **treated** immediately before severe hypoxemia causes irreversible damage to vital organs.

- **Identifying and treating** the underlying cause should be done immediately because emergency medications or surgery may be indicated. Medical treatments will vary widely depending upon the cause; for example, cardiopulmonary structural defects may require surgical repair, pulmonary edema may require diuresis, inhaled objects may require surgical removal, and infections may require aggressive antimicrobials.
- **Intravenous lines/central lines** are inserted for testing, fluids, and medications.
- **Oxygen therapy** should be initiated to attempt to reverse hypoxemia; however, if refractory hypoxemia occurs, then oxygen therapy alone will not suffice. Oxygen levels must be titrated carefully.
- **Intubation and mechanical ventilation** are frequently required to maintain adequate ventilation and oxygenation. Positive end expiratory pressure (PEEP) may be necessary with refractory hypoxemia and collapsed alveoli.
- **Respiratory status** must be monitored constantly, including arterial blood gases and vital signs.

AIR LEAK SYNDROMES

Air leak syndromes may result in significant respiratory distress. Leaks may occur spontaneously or secondary to some type of trauma (accidental, mechanical, iatrogenic) or disease. As pressure increases inside the alveoli, the alveolar wall pulls away from the perivascular sheath and subsequent alveolar rupture allows air to follow the perivascular planes and flow into adjacent areas. There are two categories:

- **Pneumothorax:**
  - Air in the pleural space causes a lung to collapse.
- **Barotrauma/volutrauma** with air in the interstitial space (usually resolve over time):
  - Pneumoperitoneum is air in the peritoneal area, including the abdomen and occasionally the scrotal sac of male infants.
  - Pneumomediastinum is air in the mediastinal area between the lungs.
  - Pneumopericardium is air in the pericardial sac that surrounds the heart.
  - Subcutaneous emphysema is air in the subcutaneous tissue planes of the chest wall.
  - Pulmonary interstitial emphysema (PIE) is air trapped in the interstitium between the alveoli.

PNEUMOTHORAX

Pneumothorax occurs when there is a leak of air into the pleural space, resulting in complete or partial collapse of a lung.

Symptoms: Vary widely depending on the cause and degree of the pneumothorax and whether or not there is an underlying disease. Symptoms include acute pleuritic pain (95%), usually on the affected side, and decreased breath sounds. In a *tension pneumothorax,* symptoms include tracheal deviation and hemodynamic compromise.

Diagnosis: Clinical findings; radiograph: 6-foot upright posterior-anterior; ultrasound may detect traumatic pneumothorax.

Treatment: Chest-tube thoracostomy with underwater seal drainage is the most common treatment for all types of pneumothorax.

- Tension pneumothorax: Immediate needle decompression and chest tube thoracostomy
- Small pneumothorax, patient stable: Oxygen administration and observation for 3-6 hours. If no increase is shown on repeat x-ray, patient may be discharged with another x-ray in 24 hours.
- Primary spontaneous pneumothorax: Catheter aspiration or chest tube thoracostomy

> **Review Video: Pneumothorax**
> Visit mometrix.com/academy and enter code: 186841

PULMONARY HYPERTENSION AND PULMONARY ARTERIAL HYPERTENSION

Pulmonary arterial hypertension (PAH) is a progressive disease of the pulmonary arteries that can severely compromise cardiovascular patients. It may involve multiple processes. Usually, the pulmonary vasculature adjusts easily to accommodate blood volume from the right ventricle. If there is increased blood flow, the low resistance causes vasodilation and vice versa. However, sometimes the pulmonary vascular bed is damaged or obstructed, and this can impair the ability to handle changing volumes of blood. In that case, an increase in flow will increase the pulmonary arterial pressure, increasing pulmonary vascular resistance (PVR). This in turn, increases pressure on the right ventricle (RV) with increased RV workload and eventually causes RV hypertrophy with displacement of the intraventricular septum and tricuspid regurgitation (cor pulmonale). Over time, this leads to right heart failure and death. Pulmonary hypertension is usually diagnosed by right-sided heart catheterization and is indicated by systolic pulmonary artery pressure >30 mmHg and mean pulmonary artery pressure >25 mmHg. Non-invasive testing may include echocardiogram to look for cardiac changes.

TYPES

Pulmonary hypertension or pulmonary arterial hypertension (PAH) may be classified as primary (idiopathic) or secondary.

- **Primary (idiopathic) PAH** may result from changes in immune responses, pulmonary emboli, sickle cell disease, collagen diseases, Raynaud's, and the use of contraceptives. The cause may be unknown or genetic.
- **Secondary PAH** may result from pulmonary vasoconstriction brought on by hypoxemia related to COPD, sleep-disordered breathing, kyphoscoliosis, obesity, smoke inhalation, altitude sickness, interstitial pneumonia, and neuromuscular disorders. It may also be caused by a decrease in pulmonary vascular bed of 50-75%, which may result from pulmonary emboli, vasculitis, tumor emboli, and interstitial lung disease, such as sarcoidosis. Primary cardiac disease, such as congenital defects in infants, and acquired disorders, such as rheumatic valve disease, mitral stenosis, and left ventricular failure may also contribute to PAH.

TREATMENT OPTIONS FOR PAH

Medical treatment for pulmonary arterial hypertension (PAH) aims to identify and treat any underlying cardiac or pulmonary disease, control symptoms, and prevent complications:

- **Oxygen therapy** may be needed, especially supplemental oxygen during exercise.
- **Calcium channel blockers** may provide vasodilation for some patients.
- **Pulmonary vascular dilators**, such as IV epoprostenol (Flolan®) and subcutaneous treprostinil sodium (Remodulin®) and oral bosentan (Tracleer®) help to control symptoms and prolong life.
- **Anticoagulants**, such as warfarin (Coumadin®) are an important part of therapy because of recurrent pulmonary emboli. Studies have shown that anticoagulation increases survival rates.
- **Diuretics**, such as furosemide (Lasix®) may be needed to relieve edema and restrict fluids, especially with right ventricular hypertrophy.

In some patients who cannot be managed adequately through medical treatment, a heart-lung transplant may be considered as the only effective treatment for long-term survival.

SLEEP APNEA
OBSTRUCTIVE SLEEP APNEA

Obstructive sleep apnea results from passive collapse of the pharynx during sleep, often associated with narrow or restricted upper airway (micrognathia, obesity, enlarged tonsils). It is most common in middle-aged overweight males and is exacerbated by ingesting alcohol or sedative drugs before sleeping. Symptoms include daytime somnolence, headache, cognitive impairment, depression, personality changes, recent increase in weight, and impotence. Patients often snore loudly with cycles of breath cessation caused by apneic periods up to 60 seconds, occurring at least 30 times a night despite continued chest wall and abdominal movements, indicating automatic attempt to breathe. ECG changes may indicate bradydysrhythmia during apnea and tachydysrhythmia when breathing resumes. Nocturnal polysomnography shows apneic periods >10 seconds (usually 20-40 seconds). There may be hypopnea with reduction of airflow. Both apneic and hypopneic periods result in reduced oxyhemoglobin saturation. If condition is severe, hypoxemia or hypercarbia may persist during waking hours.

CENTRAL SLEEP APNEA AND CENTRAL ALVEOLAR HYPOVENTILATION SYNDROME

Central sleep apnea involves apneic and hypopneic episodes without obstruction and usually results from cardiac or neurological disorders that cause impairment of ventilation. Snoring is usually mild, and individuals may complain of insomnia because they awaken frequently. Chest wall and abdominal movements do not occur during apneic periods with this breathing-related sleep disorder. Cheyne-Stokes respirations may be present (apnea, 10 to 60 seconds of hyperventilation, followed by another period of apnea). Nocturnal polysomnography shows decreased respiratory effort associated with decreased oxygen saturation.

Central alveolar hypoventilation syndrome results from impaired ventilatory control, characterized by low arterial oxygen levels and hypoventilation without apnea or hypopnea. Hypoventilation periods may persist for several minutes with sustained arterial oxygen desaturation and increased levels of carbon dioxide. This condition is often associated with obesity. Individual may complain of feeling excessively sleep or having insomnia. If condition is severe, hypoxemia or hypercarbia may persist during waking hours.

CONSERVATIVE THERAPEUTIC INTERVENTIONS FOR SLEEP APNEA

Sleep apnea intervention usually includes CPAP, although surgery may also be recommended as a last resort. However, intervention usually begins by eliminating those factors that may influence the condition. In mild cases, conservative intervention alone may be sufficient:

- Avoid drinking any alcohol in the evening as it may increase sleep apnea.
- Stop smoking as it impairs airways.
- Treat allergies, which may cause swelling and obstruction of airways.
- Control obesity by diet and exercise.
- Avoid night shift work if possible.
- Review medications with physician as some (such as tranquilizers and short acting β-blockers) may increase apnea, especially if taken in the evening.
- Change sleep position if polysomnography indicates OSA occurs only in one position (such as while supine) although this alone is usually not sufficient treatment for most people as it can be difficult to control sleep position even with bolsters and pillows.
- Bariatric surgery may be recommended if the patient is unable to lose weight and obesity is severely compromising respirations/ventilation.

THERAPEUTIC INTERVENTIONS

Potential therapies for sleep disorders include:

CPAP	Education regarding the continuous positive airway pressure (CPAP) devices should include the different types of masks available and the differences in the types of machines available: <ul><li>Bi-level PAP: Changes pressure during exhalation to facilitate breathing.</li><li>AutoPap/APAP: Has adjustable pressure rather than fixed.</li></ul> The patient should understand the importance of using a humidifier to prevent drying of mucous membranes and should understand that using the CPAP is not an option or a temporary or part-time solution but should be used with every sleep, whether at night or while napping during the daytime.
Oral/ dental devices	Some patients with mild sleep apnea may be prescribed oral or dental devices, which fit inside the mouth or are fastened around the head to open the airway during sleep. Devices include: <ul><li>Mandibular repositioning devices</li><li>Tongue retaining devices</li></ul> Patients should be cautioned to have devices fitted by professionals, such as a dentist, in order to avoid damage to the teeth, mouth, or jaw.

Endocrine

DIABETES MELLITUS TYPES 1 AND 2

Diabetes mellitus is the most common metabolic disorder. Over 6% of adults have diabetes, but only 4% of adults are diagnosed. Insulin resistance tends to increase in older adults, so there is less ability to handle glucose. Type II is more common in older adults, with incidence increasing with age.

- **Type I:** Immune-mediated form with insufficient insulin production because of the destruction of pancreatic beta cells
  - o **Symptoms** include pronounced polyuria and polydipsia, short onset, obesity or recent weight loss, and ketoacidosis present on diagnosis.
  - o **Treatment** includes insulin as needed to control blood sugar, glucose monitoring 1–4 times daily, diet with carbohydrate control, and exercise.
- **Type II:** Insulin resistant form with defect in insulin secretion
  - o **Symptoms** include long onset, obesity with no weight loss or significant weight loss, mild or absent polyuria and polydipsia, ketoacidosis or glycosuria without ketonuria, androgen-mediated problems such as hirsutism and acne (adolescents), and hypertension.
  - o **Treatment** includes diet and exercise, glucose monitoring, and oral medications.

> **Review Video: Diet, Exercise, and Medications for Diabetes**
> Visit mometrix.com/academy and enter code: 774388
>
> **Review Video: Diabetes Mellitus: Complications**
> Visit mometrix.com/academy and enter code: 996788
>
> **Review Video: Diabetes Mellitus**
> Visit mometrix.com/academy and enter code: 501396

DIABETIC KETOACIDOSIS

Diabetic ketoacidosis is a complication of type 1 diabetes mellitus, usually related to noncompliance with treatment, stress, illness, or lack of awareness of having diabetes (this event often being the first time that diabetes is diagnosed). Inadequate production of insulin results in glucose being unavailable for metabolism, so lipolysis (breakdown of fat) produces free fatty acids (FFAs) as an alternate fuel source. Glycerol is converted to ketone bodies which are used for cellular metabolism less efficiently than glucose. Excess ketone bodies are excreted in the urine (ketonuria) or exhalations. Acidosis of any type causes potassium in cells to shift to the serum. The ketone bodies lower serum pH, leading to ketoacidosis.

Symptoms include:

- Kussmaul respirations: "Ketone breath," or fruity smelling breath; progresses to CNS depression with loss of airway
- Fluid imbalance, including loss of potassium and other electrolytes from cellular death resulting in dehydration and diuresis with excess thirst
- Dangerous cardiac arrhythmias, related to potassium loss; hypotension, chest pain, tachycardia
- GI: Nausea/vomiting, abdominal pain, loss of appetite
- Neurological: malaise, confusion/lethargy progressing to coma

Diagnosis is based on:

- Labs: Blood glucose >250 mg/dL, lower Na and elevated K (switches after treatment), elevated beta-hydroxybutyrate (byproduct of ketones)
- ABG: pH <7.3, HCO_3 <18 mEq/L
- Urine: + glucose, ketones

TREATMENT AND POTENTIAL COMPLICATIONS

Treatment of DKA:

- **Fluids**: Priority is fluid resuscitation with 1-2 liters of isotonic fluids given in the first hour, up to 8 liters in the first 24 hours. Potassium will be added to the fluids when levels begin to fall.
- **Insulin**: Continuous drip IV, with/without loading dose. Will usually begin at 0.1 unit/kg/hour (5-7 units an hour generally), with a goal of decreasing blood glucose 50–75 mg/dL an hour. Blood glucose is checked every hour, and when levels are < 200 mg/dL, add dextrose to IV fluids to prevent rebound hypoglycemia.
- **Potassium**: Watch carefully, as fluids and insulin will cause rapid fall in serum levels. When K <5 mEq/L, it should be added to the IV fluids (Per liter: 20 mEq for K 4-5, 40 mEq for K 3–4). If potassium falls below 3, stop insulin drip and give 10–20 an hour until >3.5.
- **Sodium and Magnesium**: Na has an inverse relationship with potassium, and will increase as potassium falls. If sodium levels rise above 150 mEq, switch fluids to 0.45 NS. Low magnesium levels prevent potassium uptake, so replace as necessary.
- **Electrolytes**: Continue to monitor electrolytes and anion gap during ICU stay. When ABG and electrolytes normalized, transition to SQ insulin.

Potential complications include:

- Sudden electrolyte shifts (potassium) leading to catastrophic arrythmias, cerebral edema, and other complications
- Vomiting and decreased LOC leading to aspiration/ARDS
- Mechanical ventilation stops respiratory alkalosis and increases acidosis

HHNK

Hyperglycemic hyperosmolar nonketotic syndrome (HHNK) occurs in people without history of diabetes or with mild type 2 diabetes, resulting in persistent hyperglycemia leading to osmotic diuresis. Fluid shifts from intracellular to extracellular spaces to maintain osmotic equilibrium, but the increased glucosuria and dehydration results in hypernatremia and increased osmolarity. This condition is most common in those 50–70 years old and often is precipitated by an acute illness, such as a stroke, medications (thiazides), or dialysis treatments. HHNK differs from ketoacidosis because, while the insulin level is not adequate, it is high enough to prevent the breakdown of fat. Onset of symptoms often occurs over a few days. Glucose levels are often higher than those in DKA due to the gradual increase over time (often greater than 600), and the body living in a state of hyperglycemia, therefore the individual is not symptomatic until the blood glucose level is at an extreme high.

Symptoms: Polyuria, dehydration, hypotension, tachycardia, changes in mental status, seizures, hemiparesis.

Diagnosis: Increased glucose, Na, osmolality (urine and serum), BUN/Creatinine.

Treatment is similar to that for ketoacidosis:

- Insulin drip with frequent (hourly) blood sugar monitoring.
- Intravenous fluids and electrolytes.
- Correct blood glucose and other labs.

ACUTE HYPOGLYCEMIA

Acute hypoglycemia (hyperinsulinism) may result from pancreatic islet tumors or hyperplasia, increasing insulin production, or from the use of insulin to control diabetes mellitus. Hyperinsulinism can cause damage to the central nervous and cardiopulmonary systems, interfering with functioning of the brain and causing neurological impairment. Other causes may include: genetic defects (chromosome 11: short arm), severe infections, and toxic ingestion of alcohol or drugs (salicylates).

Symptoms include:

- Blood glucose <50-60 mg/dL
- Central nervous system: seizures, altered consciousness, lethargy, and poor feeding with vomiting, myoclonus, respiratory distress, diaphoresis, hypothermia, and cyanosis
- Adrenergic system: diaphoresis, tremor, tachycardia, palpitation, hunger, and anxiety

Diagnosis: Blood work, patient history, presentation.

Treatment depends on underlying cause:

- Glucose/Glucagon administration to elevate blood glucose levels
- Diazoxide (Hyperstat®) to inhibit release of insulin
- Somatostatin (Sandostatin®) to suppress insulin production
- Careful monitoring

METABOLIC SYNDROME

Metabolic syndrome is a condition that meets at least 3 of 5 diagnostic criteria :

- Hypertension (≥130/85 mmHg)
- Increased triglycerides (≥150 mg/dL)
- Decreased HDL-C (<40 mg/dL for males and <50 mg/dL for females)
- Central obesity (≥102 cm in males or ≥88 cm in females)
- Hyperglycemia (≥100 mg/dL fasting)

Metabolic syndrome is characterized by insulin resistance, which increases the risk of type 2 diabetes mellitus and atherosclerosis as insulin resistance causes macrophages to accumulate in walls of vessels. Patients are at increased risk of MI, coronary heart disease, and stroke.

Symptoms	Interventions
Many people have few symptoms initially but develop symptoms over time. • Weight gain with central obesity • Chest pain and dyspnea • Claudication • Hirsutism, acanthosis nigricans • Peripheral neuropathy • Gout	Lifestyle changes (increased exercise, less stress, weight loss, diet). Statin for high LDL. Fibrates, omega-C fatty acids for high triglycerides. Metformin for insulin resistance, type 2 diabetes. Antihypertensive (ARBs, ACEIs, BBs, diuretics). Assess for obstructive sleep apnea and treat as necessary. Aspirin prophylaxis.

CHRONIC ADRENAL INSUFFICIENCY (ADDISON'S DISEASE)

Adrenal/Adrenocortical insufficiency (Addison's disease) is caused by damage to the adrenal cortex related to a variety of causes, such as autoimmune disease or genetic disorders, but it may relate to destructive lesions or neoplasms. Without treatment the condition is life threatening.

Symptoms may be vague and the condition undiagnosed until 80–90% of the adrenal cortex has been destroyed:

- Chronic weakness and fatigue
- Abdominal distress with nausea and vomiting
- Salt or licorice craving as a result of aldosterone deficiency
- Pigmentary changes in skin and mucous membranes, hyperpigmentation
- Hypotension
- Hypoglycemia
- Recurrent seizures (more common in children)

Treatment includes hormone replacement therapy with glucocorticoids (cortisol) and mineralocorticoids (aldosterone), which may be taken orally or by monthly parenteral injections. Androgen replacement is sometimes recommended for women.

Note: During times of stress or illness, the demand for glucocorticoids may increase, and dosages up to 3 times the normal dosage may be needed to prevent an acute crisis.

> **Review Video: Addison Disease**
> Visit mometrix.com/academy and enter code: 813552

ACUTE ADRENAL INSUFFICIENCY (ADRENAL CRISIS)

Acute adrenal insufficiency (adrenal crisis) is a sudden, life-threatening condition resulting from an exacerbation of primary chronic adrenal insufficiency (Addison's disease), often precipitated by sepsis, surgical stress, adrenal hemorrhage related to septicemia, anticoagulation complications, and cortisone withdrawal related to a decreased or inadequate dose to compensate for stress. Acute adrenal insufficiency may occur in those who do not have Addison's disease, such as those who have received cortisone for various reasons, usually a minimum of 20 mg daily for at least 5 days.

Symptoms:

- Fever
- Nausea and vomiting
- Abdominal pain
- Weakness and general fatigue
- Disorientation, confusion
- Hypotensive shock
- Dehydration
- Electrolyte imbalance with hyperkalemia, hypercalcemia, hypoglycemia, and hyponatremia

Treatment:

- IV fluids in large volume
- Glucocorticoid
- 50% dextrose if indicated (hypoglycemia)
- Mineralocorticoid may be needed after intravenous solutions
- The precipitating cause must be identified and treated as well

HYPERTHYROIDISM

Hyperthyroidism (thyrotoxicosis) usually results from excess production of thyroid hormones (Graves' disease) from immunoglobulins providing abnormal stimulation of the thyroid gland. Other causes include thyroiditis and excess thyroid medications.

Symptoms vary and may be non-specific, especially in the elderly:

- Hyperexcitability
- Tachycardia (100-160) and atrial fibrillation
- Increased systolic (but not diastolic) BP
- Poor heat tolerance, skin flushed and diaphoretic
- Dry skin and pruritus (especially in the elderly)
- Hand tremor, progressive muscular weakness
- Exophthalmos (bulging eyes)
- Increased appetite and intake but weight loss

> **Review Video: Hyperthyroidism**
> Visit mometrix.com/academy and enter code: 923159
>
> **Review Video: What is Graves' Disease?**
> Visit mometrix.com/academy and enter code: 516655

Treatment includes:

- Radioactive iodine to destroy the thyroid gland. Propranolol may be used to prevent thyroid storm. Thyroid hormones are given for resultant hypothyroidism.
- Antithyroid medications, such as Propacil® or Tapazole® to block conversion of T4 to T3.

- Surgical removal of thyroid is used if patients cannot tolerate other treatments or in special circumstances, such as large goiter. Usually one-sixth of the thyroid is left in place and antithyroid medications are given before surgery.

> **Review Video: An Overview of Thyroid and Antithyroid Drugs**
> Visit mometrix.com/academy and enter code: 666133

THYROTOXIC STORM

Thyrotoxic storm is a severe type of hyperthyroidism with sudden onset, precipitated by stress such as injury or surgery, in those un-treated or inadequately treated for hyperthyroidism. If not promptly diagnosed and treated, it is fatal. Incidence has decreased with the use of antithyroid medications but can still occur with medical emergencies or pregnancy. Diagnostic findings are similar to hyperthyroidism and include increased T3 uptake and decreased TSH.

Symptoms:

- Increase in symptoms of hyperthyroidism
- Increased temperature >38.5 °C
- Tachycardia >130 with atrial fibrillation and heart failure
- Gastrointestinal disorders such as nausea, vomiting, diarrhea, and abdominal discomfort
- Altered mental status with delirium progressing to coma

Treatment:

- Controlling production of thyroid hormone through antithyroid medications such as propylthiouracil and methimazole
- Inhibiting release of thyroid hormone with iodine therapy (or lithium)
- Controlling peripheral activity of thyroid hormone with propranolol
- Fluid and electrolyte replacement
- Glucocorticoids, such as dexamethasone
- Cooling blankets
- Treatment of arrhythmias as needed with antiarrhythmics and anticoagulation

HYPOTHYROIDISM

Hypothyroidism occurs when the thyroid produces inadequate levels of thyroid hormones. Conditions may range from mild to severe myxedema. There are a number of **causes**:

- Chronic lymphocytic thyroiditis (Hashimoto's thyroiditis)
- Excessive treatment for hyperthyroidism
- Atrophy of thyroid
- Medications such as lithium and iodine compounds
- Radiation to the area of the thyroid
- Diseases that affect the thyroid such as scleroderma
- Iodine imbalances

Symptoms may include chronic fatigue, menstrual disturbances, hoarseness, subnormal temperature, low pulse rate, weight gain, thinning hair, thickening skin. Some dementia may occur with advanced conditions. Clinical findings may include increased cholesterol with associated atherosclerosis and coronary artery disease. Myxedema may be characterized by changes in respiration with hypoventilation and CO_2 retention resulting in coma.

Treatment involves hormone replacement with synthetic levothyroxine (Synthroid®) based on TSH levels, but this increases the oxygen demand of the body, so careful monitoring of cardiac status must be done during early treatment to avoid myocardial infarction while reaching euthyroid (normal) level.

Hematology

ANEMIA

Anemia occurs when there is an insufficient number of red blood cells to sufficiently oxygenate the body. As a result of the decreased level of oxygen being supplied to the organs, the body will attempt to compensate by increasing cardiac output and redistributing blood to the brain and heart. In return, the blood supply to the skin, abdominal organs, and kidneys is decreased. Anemia can occur from blood loss, increased destruction of red blood cells (hemolytic anemia), or as a result of a decreased production in red blood cells.

Signs and symptoms: Pallor, fatigue, hypotension, weakness and mental status changes. As perfusion decreases and the body attempts to compensate for the lack of oxygenation, tachycardia, chest pain, and shortness of breath may occur. In hemolytic anemias, jaundice and splenomegaly may occur as the result of the breakdown of red blood cells and the excretion of bilirubin.

Diagnosis: A complete blood count, reticulocyte count, and iron studies may be used to diagnose anemia.

Treatment: The treatment of anemia is focused on treating the underlying cause. Parenteral iron may be given for patients with iron deficiency anemias caused from chronic blood loss, or inadequate iron intake or absorption. Blood transfusions are used to treat patients with active bleeding as well as those patients who are displaying significant clinical symptoms. Erythropoietin stimulating proteins may also be utilized to decrease the need for a transfusion.

SICKLE CELL DISEASE

Sickle cell disease is a recessive genetic disorder of chromosome 11, causing hemoglobin to be defective so that red blood cells (RBCs) are sickle-shaped and inflexible, resulting in their accumulating in small vessels and causing painful blockage. While normal RBCs survive 120 days, sickled cells may survive only 10-20 days, stressing the bone marrow that cannot produce fast enough and resulting in severe anemia. There are 5 variations of sickle cell disease, with sickle cell anemia the most severe. Different types of crises occur (aplastic, hemolytic, vaso-occlusive, and sequestrating), which can cause infarctions in organs, severe pain, damage to organs, and rapid enlargement of liver and spleen. Complications include anemia, acute chest syndrome, congestive heart failure, strokes, delayed growth, infections, pulmonary hypertension, liver and kidney disorders, retinopathy, seizures, and osteonecrosis. Sickle cell disease occurs almost exclusively in African Americans in the United States, with 8-10% carriers.

> **Review Video: Sickle Cell Disease**
> Visit mometrix.com/academy and enter code: 603869

TREATMENT

Treatment for sickle cell disease includes:

- **Prophylactic penicillin** for children from 2 months to 5 years to prevent pneumonia
- **IV fluids** to prevent dehydration
- **Analgesics** (morphine) during painful crises
- **Folic acid** for anemia
- **Oxygen** for congestive heart failure or pulmonary disease

- **Blood transfusions** with chelation therapy to remove excess iron OR erythropheresis, in which red cells are removed and replaced with healthy cells, either autologous or from a donor
- **Hematopoietic stem cells transplantation** is the only curative treatment, but immunosuppressive drugs must be used and success rates are only about 85%, so the procedure is only used on those at high risk. It requires ablation of bone marrow, placing the patient at increased risk.
- **Partial chimerism** uses a mixture of the donor and the recipient's bone marrow stem cells and does not require ablation of bone marrow. It is showing good success.

POLYCYTHEMIA VERA

Polycythemia vera is a condition in which there is abnormal production of blood cells in the bone marrow. Erythrocytes (red blood cells) are primarily affected. The disease is more common in men older than 40 years. Polycythemia may be primary or secondary, related to conditions causing hypoxia. The blood increases in viscosity, resulting in a number of **symptoms**:

- Dizziness, headache, weakness, and fatigue
- Dyspnea, especially when supine
- Flushing of skin, blue-tinged skin discoloration, and red lesions
- Itching after warm bath
- Left upper abdominal fullness and splenomegaly
- Phlebitis from blood clots
- Vision disturbances
- Complications include stroke, hemorrhage, and heart failure

Diagnosis includes CBC with differential, chemistry panel, bone marrow biopsy, and Vitamin B_{12} level. Red cell mass will be more than 25% above normal.

Treatment includes:

- **Phlebotomy** to remove 500 mL (lesser amounts for children) of blood to decrease blood viscosity, repeated weekly until hematocrit stable (less than 45%)
- Referral for **chemotherapy** (hydroxyurea) to suppress marrow production
- **Interferon** to decrease need for phlebotomy

VON WILLEBRAND DISEASE

Von Willebrand disease is a group of congenital bleeding disorders (inherited from either parent) affecting 1-2% of the population, associated with deficiency or lack of von Willebrand factor (vWF), a glycoprotein that is synthesized, stored, and secreted by vascular endothelial cells. This protein interacts with thrombocytes to create a clot and prevent hemorrhage; however, with von Willebrand disease, this clotting mechanism is impaired. There are three types:

- **Type I**: Low levels of vWF and also sometimes factor VIII (dominant inheritance)
- **Type II**: Abnormal vWF (subtypes a, b) may increase or decrease clotting (dominant inheritance)
- **Type III**: Absence of vWF and less than 10% factor VIII (recessive inheritance)

Symptoms vary in severity and include bruising, menorrhagia, recurrent epistaxis, and hemorrhage.

Treatment includes:

- **Desmopressin acetate** parenterally or nasally to stimulate production of clotting factor (mild cases)
- **Severe bleeding**: factor VIII concentrates with vWF, such as Humate-P

HEMOPHILIA

Hemophilia is an inherited disorder in which the person lacks adequate clotting factors. There are three types:

- **Type A**: lack of clotting factor VIII (90% of cases)
- **Type B**: lack of clotting factor IX
- **Type C**: lack of clotting factor XI (affects both sexes, rarely occurs in the United States)

Both Type A and B are usually X-linked disorders, affecting only males. The severity of the disease depends on the amount of clotting factor in the blood.

Symptoms:

- Bleeding with severe trauma or stress (mild cases)
- Unexplained bruises, bleeding, swelling, joint pain
- Spontaneous hemorrhage (severe cases), often in the joints but can be anywhere in the body
- Epistaxis, mucosal bleeding
- First symptoms often occur during infancy when the child becomes active, resulting in frequent bruises

Treatment:

- Desmopressin acetate parenterally or nasally to stimulate production of clotting factor (mild cases)
- Infusions of clotting factor from donated blood or recombinant clotting factors (genetically engineered), utilizing guidelines for dosing
- Infusions of plasma (Type C)

DISSEMINATED INTRAVASCULAR COAGULATION

PATHOLOGY

Disseminated intravascular coagulation (DIC) (consumption coagulopathy) is a secondary disorder that is triggered by another disorder such as trauma, congenital heart disease, necrotizing enterocolitis, sepsis, and severe viral infections. DIC triggers both coagulation and hemorrhage through a complex series of events. Trauma causes tissue factor (transmembrane glycoprotein) to enter the circulation and bind with coagulation factors, triggering the coagulation cascade. This stimulates thrombin to convert fibrinogen to fibrin, causing aggregation and destruction of platelets and forming clots that can be disseminated throughout the intravascular system. These clots increase in size as platelets adhere to the clots, causing blockage of both the microvascular systems and larger vessels, which can result in ischemia and necrosis. Clot formation triggers fibrinolysis and plasmin to breakdown fibrin and fibrinogen, causing the destruction of clotting factors and resulting in hemorrhage. Both processes, clotting and hemorrhage, continue at the same time, placing the patient at high risk for death, even with treatment.

SYMPTOMS AND TREATMENT

The onset of symptoms of DIC may be very rapid or be a slower chronic progression from a disease. Those who develop the chronic manifestation of the disease usually have fewer acute symptoms and may slowly develop ecchymosis or bleeding wounds.

Symptoms include:

- Bleeding from surgical or venous puncture sites
- Evidence of GI bleeding with distention, bloody diarrhea
- Hypotension and acute symptoms of shock
- Petechiae and purpura with extensive bleeding into the tissues
- Laboratory abnormalities:
  - Prolonged prothrombin and partial prothrombin times
  - Decreased platelet counts and fragmented RBCs
  - Decreased fibrinogen

Treatment includes:

- Identifying and treating underlying cause
- Massive blood transfusion protocol; replacement of blood products, such as platelets and fresh frozen plasma
- Anticoagulation therapy (heparin) to increase clotting time
- Cryoprecipitate to increase fibrinogen levels
- Coagulation inhibitors and coagulation factors

THROMBOCYTOPENIA

Thrombocytopenia is a deficiency of circulating platelets in the blood. It can be caused by a decrease in the production of platelets from the bone marrow or an increase in destruction of platelets. Thrombocytopenia may also be caused from the use of heparin. Heparin induced thrombocytopenia can occur after heparin therapy (average 4-14 days post therapy) and is characterized by a decrease in platelet count to less than 50% of baseline or the occurrence of an unexplained thrombolytic event. A decreased production of platelets within the bone marrow can occur as a result of malignancy, bone marrow failure, infection, alcohol abuse, or a nutritional deficiency. An increase in the destruction of platelets may occur in disseminated intravascular coagulation, vasculitis, thrombotic thrombocytopenic purpura, sepsis, or idiopathic thrombocytopenic purpura.

Signs and symptoms: Signs and symptoms may include petechiae, ecchymosis, bleeding from the mouth or gums, epistaxis, pallor, weakness, fatigue, splenomegaly, blood in the urine or stool, and jaundice.

Diagnosis: Physical exam and lab studies including complete blood count, partial thromboplastin time and prothrombin time may be used to diagnosis thrombocytopenia. A bone marrow biopsy may be indicated to determine the cause of the decreased production of platelets.

Treatment: Treatment of thrombocytopenia involves identifying and treating the underlying cause. Medications that decrease the platelet count should be held. Platelet transfusions may be administered to patients with extremely low counts (less than 50,000) or if spontaneous bleeding occurs. Platelet transfusions are contraindicated in patients with thrombotic thrombocytopenia purpura.

ITP

The autoimmune disorder **idiopathic thrombocytopenic purpura (ITP)** causes an immune response to platelets, resulting in decreased platelet counts. ITP affects primarily children and young women although it can occur at any age. The acute form primarily occurs in children, but the chronic form affects primarily adults. Platelet counts are usually 150,000–400,000 per mcL. With ITP, platelet levels are less than 100,000. Maintaining a platelet count of at least 30,000 is necessary to prevent intracranial hemorrhage, the primary concern. The cause of ITP is unclear and may be precipitated by viral infection, sulfa drugs, and conditions, such as lupus erythematosus. ITP is usually not life threatening and can be controlled. **Symptoms** include:

- Bruising and petechiae with hematoma in some cases
- Epistaxis
- Increased menstrual flow in post-puberty females

Treatment includes:

- Corticosteroids to depress immune response and increase platelet count
- Splenectomy may be indicated for chronic conditions
- Platelet transfusions
- Avoiding aspirin, ibuprofen, or other NSAIDs

HITTS

Heparin-induced thrombocytopenia and thrombosis syndrome (HITTS) occurs in patients receiving heparin for anticoagulation. There are two types:

- **Type I** is a transient condition occurring within a few days and causing depletion of platelets (<100,000 mm³), but heparin may be continued as the condition usually resolves without intervention.
- **Type II** is an autoimmune reaction to heparin that occurs in 3–5% of those receiving unfractionated heparin and also occurs with low-molecular-weight heparin. It is characterized by low platelets (<50,000 mm³) that are ≥50% below baseline. Onset is 5–14 days but can occur within hours of heparinization. Death rates are <30%. Heparin-antibody complexes form and release platelet factor 4 (PF4), which attracts heparin molecules and adheres to platelets and endothelial lining, stimulating thrombin and platelet clumping. This puts the patient at risk for thrombosis and vessel occlusion rather than hemorrhage, causing stroke, myocardial infarction, and limb ischemia with symptoms associated with the site of thrombosis. Treatment includes:
  - Discontinuation of heparin
  - Direct thrombin inhibitors (lepirudin, argatroban)
  - Monitor for signs/symptoms of thrombus/embolus

Neurology

HEMORRHAGIC STROKES

Hemorrhagic strokes account for about 20% of all strokes and result from a ruptured cerebral artery, causing not only a lack of oxygen and nutrients but also edema that causes widespread pressure and damage:

- **Intracerebral** is bleeding into the substance of the brain from an artery in the central lobes, basal ganglia, pons, or cerebellum. Intracerebral hemorrhage usually results from atherosclerotic degenerative changes, hypertension, brain tumors, anticoagulation therapy, or use of illicit drugs, such as cocaine.
- **Intracranial aneurysm** occurs with ballooning cerebral artery ruptures, most commonly at the Circle of Willis.
- **Arteriovenous malformation**. Rupture of AVMs can cause brain attack in young adults.
- **Subarachnoid hemorrhage** is bleeding in the space between the meninges and brain, resulting from aneurysm, AVM, or trauma. This type of hemorrhage compresses brain tissue.

Treatment includes: The patient may need airway protection/artificial ventilation if neurologic compromise is severe. Blood pressure is lowered to control rate of bleeding but with caution to avoid hypotension and resulting cerebral ischemia (Goal – CPP >70). Sedation can lower ICP and blood pressure, and seizure prophylaxis will be indicated as blood irritates the cerebral cells. An intraventricular catheter may be used in ICP management; correct any clotting disorders if identified.

ISCHEMIA STROKES

Strokes (brain attacks, cerebrovascular accidents) result when there is interruption of the blood flow to an area of the brain. The two basic types are ischemic and hemorrhagic. About 80% are **ischemic**, resulting from blockage of an artery supplying the brain:

- **Thrombosis** in a large artery, usually resulting from atherosclerosis, may block circulation to a large area of the brain. It is most common in the elderly and may occur suddenly or after episodes of transient ischemic attacks.
- **Lacunar infarct** (a penetrating thrombosis in a small artery) is most common in those with diabetes mellitus and/or hypertension.
- **Embolism** travels through the arterial system and lodges in the brain, most commonly in the left middle cerebral artery. An embolism may be cardiogenic, resulting from cardiac arrhythmia or surgery. An embolism usually occurs rapidly with no warning signs.
- **Cryptogenic** has no identifiable cause.

Medical management of ischemic strokes with tissue plasminogen activator (tPA) (Activase®), the primary treatment, should be initiated within 3 hours (or up to 4.5 hours if inclusion criteria are met):

- **Thrombolytic,** such as tPA, which is produced by recombinant DNA and is used to dissolve fibrin clots. It is given intravenously (0.9 mg/kg up to 90 mg) with 10% injected as an initial bolus and the rest over the next hour.
- **Antihypertensives** if MAP >130 mmHg or systolic BP >220
- **Cooling** to reduce hyperthermia

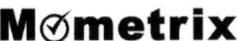

- **Osmotic diuretics** (mannitol), hypertonic saline, loop diuretics (Lasix®), and/or corticosteroids (dexamethasone) to decrease cerebral edema and intracranial pressure
- **Aspirin/anticoagulation** may be used with embolism
- Monitor and treat hyperglycemia
- **Surgical Intervention:** Used when other treatment fails, may go in through artery and manually remove the clot

SYMPTOMS OF BRAIN ATTACKS IN RELATION TO AREA OF BRAIN AFFECTED

Brain attacks most commonly occur in the right or left hemisphere, but the exact location and the extent of brain damage from a brain attack affects the type of presenting symptoms. If the frontal area of either side is involved, there tends to be memory and learning deficits. Some symptoms are common to specific areas and help to identify the area involved:

- **Right hemisphere**: This results in left paralysis or paresis and a left visual field deficit that may cause spatial and perceptual disturbances, so people may have difficulty judging distance. Fine motor skills may be impacted, resulting in trouble dressing or handling tools. People may become impulsive and exhibit poor judgment, often denying impairment. Left-sided neglect (lack of perception of things on the left side) may occur. Difficulty following directions, short-term memory loss, and depression are also common. Language skills usually remain intact.
- **Left hemisphere**: Results in right paralysis or paresis and a right visual field defect. Depression is common and people often exhibit slow, cautious behavior, requiring repeated instruction and reinforcement for simple tasks. Short-term memory loss and difficulty learning new material or understanding generalizations is common. Difficulty with mathematics, reading, writing, and reasoning may occur. Aphasia (expressive, receptive, or global) is common.
- **Brain stem**: Because the brain stem controls respiration and cardiac function, a brain attack in the brain stem frequently causes death, but those who survive may have a number of problems, including respiratory and cardiac abnormalities. Strokes may involve motor or sensory impairment or both.
- **Cerebellum**: This area controls balance and coordination. Brain attacks in the cerebellum are rare but may result in ataxia, nausea and vomiting, and headaches and dizziness or vertigo.

TIA

Transient ischemic attacks (TIAs) from small clots cause similar but short-lived (minutes to hours) symptoms. Emergent treatment includes placing patient in semi-Fowlers or Fowler's position and administering oxygen. The patient may require oral suctioning if secretions pool. The patient's circulation, airway, and breathing should be assessed and IV access line placed. Thrombolytic therapy to dissolve blood clots should be administered within 1 to 3 hours. While a patient can recover fully from a TIA, they should be educated, because having a TIA increases an individual's risk for a stroke.

> **Review Video: Overview of Strokes**
> Visit mometrix.com/academy and enter code: 310572

Renal

ACUTE TUBULAR NECROSIS

Acute tubular necrosis (ATN) occurs when a hypoxic condition causes renal ischemia that damages tubular cells of the glomeruli so they are unable to adequately filter the urine, leading to acute renal failure. Causes include hypotension, hyperbilirubinemia, sepsis, surgery (especially cardiac or vascular), and birth complications. ATN may result from nephrotoxic injury related to obstruction or drugs, such as chemotherapy, acyclovir, and antibiotics, such as sulfonamides and streptomycin. Symptoms may be non-specific initially and can include life-threatening complications.

Symptoms include:

- Lethargy
- Nausea and vomiting
- Hypovolemia with low cardiac output and generalized vasodilation
- Fluid and electrolyte imbalance leading to hypertension, CNS abnormalities, metabolic acidosis, arrhythmias, edema, and congestive heart failure
- Uremia leading to destruction of platelets and bleeding, neurological deficits, and disseminated intravascular coagulopathy (DIC)
- Infections, including pericarditis and sepsis

Treatment includes:

- Identifying and treating underlying cause, discontinuing nephrotoxic agents
- Supportive care
- Loop diuretics (in some cases), such as Lasix®
- Antibiotics for infection (can include pericarditis and sepsis)
- Kidney dialysis

ACUTE KIDNEY INJURY

Acute kidney injury (AKI), previously known as acute renal failure, is an acute disruption of kidney function that results in decreased renal perfusion, a decrease in glomerular filtration rate and a buildup of metabolic waste products (azotemia). Azotemia is the accumulation of urea, creatinine and other nitrogen containing end products into the bloodstream. The regulation of fluid volume, electrolyte balance and acid base balance is also affected. The causes of acute kidney injury are divided into pre-renal (caused by a decrease in perfusion), intrarenal or intrinsic (occurring within the kidney) and post-renal (caused by the inadequate drainage of urine). Acute kidney injury is common in hospitalized patients and even more common in critically ill patients, carrying a mortality rate of 50-80%. Risk factors for acute kidney injury include advanced age, the presence of co-morbid conditions, pre-existing kidney disease and a diagnosis of sepsis.

Signs and symptoms: Malaise, fatigue, lethargy, confusion, weakness, change in urine color, change in urine volume, and flank pain.

Diagnosis: Urinalysis, serum BUN and creatinine levels, renal ultrasound, CT or MRI and renal biopsy.

Treatment: The treatment of acute kidney injury is based on the underlying cause. Treatment options may include fluid and electrolyte replacement, diuretic therapy, fluid restriction, renal diet, and low dose dopamine to increase renal perfusion. Hemodialysis may also be necessary in patients with acute kidney injury.

Review Video: Acute Kidney Injury (AKI)
Visit mometrix.com/academy and enter code: 780321

CHRONIC KIDNEY DISEASE

Chronic kidney disease (CKD) occurs when the kidneys are unable to filter and excrete wastes, concentrate urine, and maintain electrolyte balance because of hypoxic conditions, kidney disease, or obstruction in the urinary tract. It results first in azotemia (increase in nitrogenous waste in the blood) and then in uremia (nitrogenous wastes cause toxic symptoms). When >50% of the functional renal capacity is destroyed, the kidneys can no longer carry out necessary functions, and progressive deterioration begins over months or years. Symptoms are often non-specific in the beginning, with loss of appetite and energy.

Symptoms and complications are as follows:

- Weight loss
- Headaches, muscle cramping, general malaise
- Increased bruising and dry or itchy skin
- Increased BUN and creatinine
- Sodium and fluid retention with edema
- Hyperkalemia
- Metabolic acidosis
- Calcium and phosphorus depletion, resulting in altered bone metabolism, pain, and retarded growth
- Anemia with decreased production on RBCs. Increased risk of infection
- Uremic syndrome

Treatment includes:

- Supportive/symptomatic therapy
- Dialysis and transplantation
- Diet control: low protein, salt, potassium, and phosphorus
- Fluid limitations
- Calcium and vitamin supplementation
- Phosphate binders

UREMIC SYNDROME

Uremic syndrome is a number of disorders that can occur with end-stage renal disease and renal failure, usually after multiple metabolic failures and decrease in creatinine clearance to <10 mL/min. There is compromise of all normal functions of the kidney: fluid balance, electrolyte balance, acid-base homeostasis, hormone production, and elimination of wastes. Metabolic abnormalities related to uremia include:

- **Decreased RBC production**: The kidney is unable to produce adequate erythropoietin in the peritubular cells, resulting in anemia, which is usually normocytic and normochromic. Parathyroid hormone levels may increase, causing calcification of the bone marrow, causing hypoproliferative anemia as RBC production is suppressed.

- **Platelet abnormalities**: Decreased platelet count, increased turnover, and reduced adhesion leads to bleeding disorders.
- **Metabolic acidosis**: The tubular cells are unable to regulate acid-base metabolism, and phosphate, sulfuric, hippuric, and lactic acids increase, leading to congestive heart failure and weakness.
- **Hyperkalemia**: The nephrons cannot excrete adequate amounts of potassium. Some drugs, such as diuretics that spare potassium may aggravate the condition.
- **Renal bone disease**: Decreased calcium, elevated phosphate, elevated parathyroid hormone, decreased utilization of vitamin D lead to demineralization. In some cases, calcium and phosphate are deposited in other tissues (metastatic calcification).
- **Multiple endocrine disorders**: Thyroid hormone production is decreased and abnormalities in reproductive hormones may result in infertility/impotence. Males have decreased testosterone but elevated estrogen and LH. Females experience irregular cycles, lack of ovulation and menses. Insulin production may increase but with decreased clearance, resulting in episodes of hypoglycemia or decreased hyperglycemia in those who are diabetic.
- **Cardiovascular disorders**: Left ventricular hypertrophy is most common, but fluid retention may cause congestive heart failure and electrolyte imbalances, dysrhythmias. Pericarditis, exacerbation of valvular disorders, and pericardial effusions may occur.
- **Anorexia and malnutrition**: Nausea and poor appetite contribute to hypoalbuminemia, sometimes exacerbated by restrictive diets.

ELECTROLYTE IMBALANCES

SODIUM

Sodium (**Na**) regulates fluid volume, osmolality, acid-base balance, and activity in the muscles, nerves, and myocardium. It is the primary **cation** (positive ion) in extracellular fluid (ECF), necessary to maintain ECF levels that are needed for tissue perfusion:

- Normal range: 135-145 mEq/L
- Hyponatremia: <135 mEq/L
- Hypernatremia: >145 mEq/L

Hyponatremia may result from inadequate sodium intake, excess sodium loss through diarrhea, vomiting, or NG suctioning, or illness, such as severe burns, fever, SIADH, and ketoacidosis.

- **Symptoms**: Irritability to lethargy and alterations in consciousness, cerebral edema with seizures and coma, dyspnea to respiratory failure.
- **Treatment**: Identify and treat the underlying cause and provide Na replacement.

Hypernatremia may result from renal disease, diabetes insipidus, and fluid depletion.

- **Symptoms**: Irritability to lethargy to confusion to coma; seizures; flushing; muscle weakness and spasms; thirst.
- **Treatment**: Identify and treat the underlying cause, monitor Na levels carefully, and give IV fluid replacement.

POTASSIUM

Potassium (**K**) is the primary **electrolyte** in intracellular fluid (ICF), with about 98% inside cells and only 2% in ECF, although this small amount is important for neuromuscular activity. Potassium influences activity of the skeletal and cardiac muscles. Its level is dependent upon adequate renal functioning because 80% is excreted through the kidneys and 20% through the bowels and sweat:

- Normal range: 3.5-5.5 mEq/L
- Hypokalemia: <3.5 mEq/L. Critical value: <2.5 mEq/L
- Hyperkalemia: >5.5 mEq/L. Critical value: >6.5 mEq/L

A healthy NPO patient will need about 40 mEq of K per day to maintain serum K levels. Expect alterations in renal disease and other disease processes.

Hypokalemia is caused by alkalosis, decreased intake associated with starvation, nephritis, and loss of potassium through diarrhea, vomiting, gastric suction, and diuresis.

- **Symptoms**: Lethargy and weakness; nausea and vomiting; paresthesia and tetany; muscle cramps with hyporeflexia; hypotension; dysrhythmias with EKG changes: PVCs or flattened T-waves.
- **Treatment**: Treatment involves identifying and treating the underlying cause and replacing K. When possible, oral replacement is preferable to IV, as it allows slower adjustment of K levels. When given IV, K should be given no faster than 20 mEq/hour via central line if possible. If given peripherally, 10 mEq/hour is preferable for patient comfort.

Hyperkalemia is caused by renal disease, adrenal insufficiency, metabolic acidosis, severe dehydration, burns, hemolysis, and trauma. It rarely occurs without renal disease but may be induced by treatment (such as NSAIDs and potassium-sparing diuretics). Untreated renal failure results in reduced excretion. Those with Addison's disease and deficient adrenal hormones suffer sodium loss that results in potassium retention.

- **Symptoms**: The primary symptoms relate to the effect on the cardiac muscle: ventricular arrhythmias with increasing changes in EKG lead to cardiac and respiratory arrest, weakness with ascending paralysis and hyperreflexia, diarrhea, and increasing confusion.
- **Treatment**: Treatment includes identifying the underlying cause and discontinuing sources of increased K. Calcium gluconate to decrease cardiac effects. Sodium bicarbonate, insulin, and hypertonic dextrose shift K into the cells temporarily. Cation exchange resin (Kayexalate®) to decrease K. Peritoneal dialysis or hemodialysis to remove excess K.

Note: When a tourniquet is on, a patient opening and closing their hand can lead to falsely elevated K levels.

CALCIUM

More than 99% of calcium (**Ca**) is in the skeletal system with 1% in serum, but it is important for transmitting nerve impulses and regulating muscle contraction and relaxation, including the myocardium. Calcium activates enzymes that stimulate chemical reactions and has a role in the coagulation of blood:

- Normal range: 8.2-10.2 mg/dL
- Hypocalcemia: <8.2. Critical value: <7 mg/dL
- Hypercalcemia: >10.2 mg/dL. Critical value: >12 mg/dL

Hypercalcemia may be caused by acidosis, kidney disease, hyperparathyroidism, prolonged immobilization, and malignancies. Crisis carries a 50% mortality rate.

- **Symptoms**: Increasing muscle weakness with hypotonicity; anorexia; nausea and vomiting; constipation; bradycardia and cardiac arrest.
- **Treatment**: Identify and treat underlying cause, loop diuretics, IV fluids, phosphate.

Hypocalcemia may be caused by damage to the parathyroid resulting in hypoparathyroidism (directly decreasing calcium production), vitamin D resistance or inadequacy, or liver/kidney disease.

- **Symptoms**: Muscle cramping or spasms; seizures; numbness or tingling of the feet, hands, or lips; tetany if severe.
- **Treatment**: Identify and treat underlying cause, replace calcium by administering IV calcium gluconate in acute circumstances or increasing oral Vitamin D and calcium in chronic cases.

PHOSPHORUS

Phosphorus, or phosphate, (PO_4) is necessary for neuromuscular and red blood cell function, the maintenance of acid-base balance, and provides structure for teeth and bones. About 85% is in the bones, 14% in soft tissue, and <1% in ECF.

- Normal range: 2.4-4.5 mEq/L
- Hypophosphatemia: <2.4mEq/L
- Hyperphosphatemia: >4.5 mEq/L

Hypophosphatemia occurs with severe protein-calorie malnutrition, hyperventilation, severe burns, diabetic ketoacidosis, and excess antacids with magnesium, calcium, or aluminum.

- **Symptoms**: Irritability, tremors, seizures to coma; hemolytic anemia; decreased myocardial function; respiratory failure.
- **Treatment**: Identify and treat underlying cause and replace phosphorus.

Hyperphosphatemia occurs with renal failure, hypoparathyroidism, excessive intake, neoplastic disease, diabetic ketoacidosis, muscle necrosis, and chemotherapy.

- **Symptoms**: Tachycardia; muscle cramping; hyperreflexia and tetany; nausea and diarrhea.
- **Treatment**: Identify and treat underlying cause, correct hypocalcemia, and provide antacids and dialysis.

MAGNESIUM

Magnesium (**Mg**) is the second most common intracellular electrolyte (after potassium) and activates many intracellular enzyme systems. Mg is important for carbohydrate and protein metabolism, neuromuscular function, and cardiovascular function, producing vasodilation and directly affecting the peripheral arterial system:

- Normal range: 1.7-2.2 mg/dL
- Hypomagnesemia critical value: <1.2 mg/dL
- Hypermagnesemia critical value: >4.9 mg/dL

Hypomagnesemia occurs with chronic diarrhea, chronic renal disease, chronic pancreatitis, excess diuretic or laxative use, hyperthyroidism, hypoparathyroidism, severe burns, and diaphoresis.

- **Symptoms:** Neuromuscular excitability or tetany; confusion, headaches, dizziness; seizure and coma; tachycardia with ventricular arrhythmias; respiratory depression.
- **Treatment:** Identify and treat underlying cause, provide magnesium replacement. IV magnesium is a vasodilator, 2 g over 60 mins.

Hypermagnesemia occurs with renal failure or inadequate renal function, diabetic ketoacidosis, hypothyroidism, and Addison's disease.

- **Symptoms:** Muscle weakness, seizures, and dysphagia with decreased gag reflex; tachycardia with hypotension.
- **Treatment:** Identify and treat underlying cause, IV hydration with calcium, and dialysis.

> **Review Video: Fluid and Electrolyte Balance**
> Visit mometrix.com/academy and enter code: 384389

Multisystem

RANGE OF SEVERE INFECTION

There are a number of terms used to refer to severe infections which are often used interchangeably. It is important to know these terms to properly perform the continuum of care.

- **Bacteremia** is the presence of bacteria in the blood without systemic infection.
- **Septicemia** is a systemic infection caused by pathogens (usually bacteria or fungi) present in the blood.
- **Systemic inflammatory response syndrome** (SIRS) is a generalized inflammatory response affecting many organ systems. It may be caused by infectious or non-infectious agents, such as trauma, burns, adrenal insufficiency, pulmonary embolism, and drug overdose. If an infectious agent is identified or suspected, SIRS is an aspect of sepsis. Infective agents include a wide range of bacteria and fungi, including *Streptococcus pneumoniae* and *Staphylococcus aureus*. SIRS includes 2 of the following:
  - Elevated (>38 °C) or subnormal rectal temperature (<36 °C)
  - Tachypnea or $PaCO_2$ <32 mmHg
  - Tachycardia
  - Leukocytosis (>12,000) or leukopenia (<4000)
- **Sepsis** is the presence of infection either locally or systemically in which there is a generalized life-threatening inflammatory response (SIRS). It includes all the indications for SIRS as well as one of the following:
  - Changes in mental status
  - Hypoxemia without preexisting pulmonary disease
  - Elevation in plasma lactate
  - Decreased urinary output <5 mL/kg/hr for ≥1 hour
- **Severe sepsis** includes both indications of SIRS and sepsis as well as indications of increasing organ dysfunction with inadequate perfusion and/or hypotension.
- **Septic shock** is a progression from severe sepsis in which refractory hypotension occurs despite treatment. There may be indications of lactic acidosis.
- **Multi-organ dysfunction syndrome** (MODS) is the most common cause of sepsis-related death. Cardiac function becomes depressed, acute respiratory distress syndrome (ARDS) may develop, and renal failure may follow acute tubular necrosis or cortical necrosis. Thrombocytopenia appears in about 30% of those affected and may result in disseminated intravascular coagulation (DIC). Liver damage and bowel necrosis may occur.

SHOCK

There are a number of different types of shock, but there are general characteristics that they have in common. In all types of shock, there is a marked decrease in tissue perfusion related to hypotension, so that there is insufficient oxygen delivered to the tissues and inadequate removal of cellular waste products, causing injury to tissue:

- Hypotension (systolic below 90 mmHg); this may be somewhat higher (110 mmHg) in those who are initially hypertensive
- Decreased urinary output (<0.5 mL/kg/hr), especially marked in hypovolemic shock
- Metabolic acidosis
- Peripheral/cutaneous vasoconstriction/vasodilation resulting in cool, clammy skin
- Alterations in level of consciousness

Types of shock are as follows:

- **Distributive:** Preload decreased, CO increased, SVR decreased
- **Cardiogenic:** Preload increased, CO decreased, SVR increased
- **Hypovolemic:** Preload decreased, CO decreased, SVR increased

SEPTIC SHOCK

Septic shock is caused by toxins produced by bacteria and cytokines that the body produces in response to severe infection, resulting in a complex syndrome of disorders. **Symptoms** are wide-ranging:

- **Initial:** Hyper- or hypothermia, increased temperature (>38 °C) with chills, tachycardia with increased pulse pressure, tachypnea, alterations in mental status (dullness), hypotension, hyperventilation with respiratory alkalosis ($PaCO_2$ ≤30 mmHg), increased lactic acid, unstable BP, and dehydration with increased urinary output
- **Cardiovascular:** Myocardial depression and dysrhythmias
- **Respiratory:** Acute respiratory distress syndrome (ARDS)
- **Renal:** Acute kidney injury (AKI) with decreased urinary output and increased BUN
- **Hepatic:** Jaundice and liver dysfunction with an increase in transaminase, alkaline phosphatase, and bilirubin
- **Hematologic:** Mild or severe blood loss (from mucosal ulcerations), neutropenia or neutrophilia, decreased platelets, and DIC
- **Endocrine:** Hyperglycemia, hypoglycemia (rare)
- **Skin:** Cellulitis, erysipelas, and fasciitis, acrocyanotic and necrotic peripheral lesions

DIAGNOSIS AND TREATMENT

Septic shock is most common in newborns, those >50, and those who are immunocompromised. There is no specific test to confirm a diagnosis of septic shock, so **diagnosis** is based on clinical findings and tests that evaluate hematologic, infectious, and metabolic states: Lactic acid, CBC, DIC panel, electrolytes, liver function tests, BUN, creatinine, blood glucose, ABGs, urinalysis, ECG, radiographs, blood and urine cultures.

Treatment must be aggressive and includes:

- Oxygen and endotracheal intubation as necessary
- IV access with 2-large bore catheters and central venous line
- Rapid fluid administration at 0.5L NS or isotonic crystalloid every 5-10 minutes as needed (to 4-6 L)
- Monitoring urinary output to optimal >30 mL/hr (>0.5-1 mL/kg/hr)
- Inotropic or vasoconstrictive agents (dopamine, dobutamine, norepinephrine) if no response to fluids or fluid overload
- Empiric IV antibiotic therapy (usually with 2 broad spectrum antibiotics for both gram-positive and gram-negative bacteria) until cultures return and antibiotics may be changed
- Hemodynamic and laboratory monitoring
- Removing source of infection (abscess, catheter)

DISTRIBUTIVE SHOCK

Distributive shock occurs with adequate blood volume but inadequate intravascular volume because of arterial/venous dilation that results in decreased vascular tone and hypoperfusion of internal organs. Cardiac output may be normal or blood may pool, decreasing cardiac output.

Distributive shock may result from anaphylactic shock, septic shock, neurogenic shock, and drug ingestions.

Symptoms include:

- Hypotension (systolic <90 mmHg or <40 mmHg below normal), tachypnea, tachycardia (>90) (may be lower if patient receiving β-blockers)
- Hypoxemia
- Skin initially warm, later hypoperfused
- Hyper- or hypothermia (>38 °C or <36 °C)
- Alterations in mentation
- Decreased urinary output
- Symptoms related to underlying cause

Treatment includes:

- Treating underlying cause while stabilizing hemodynamics
- Oxygen with endotracheal intubation if necessary
- Rapid fluid administration at 0.25-0.5 L NS or isotonic crystalloid every 5-10 minutes as needed to 2-3 L
- Vasoconstrictive and inotropic agents (dopamine, dobutamine, norepinephrine) if necessary, for patients with profound hypotension

CARDIOGENIC SHOCK

In cardiogenic shock, the heart fails to pump enough blood to provide adequate circulation and oxygen to the body. The primary cause of cardiogenic shock is acute myocardial infarction, especially an anterior wall MI. Other causes include papillary muscle/ventricular septal rupture, pericarditis/myocarditis, prolonged tachyarrhythmia, and hypotensive medications.

Signs/Symptoms: Hypotension, altered mental status secondary to decreased cerebral circulation, oliguria, tachypnea or tachycardia, cool extremities, jugular venous distension, and pulmonary edema possible.

Diagnosis: ABGs: metabolic acidosis, hypoxia, hypocapnia; lactic acidosis, BNP, BUN and K elevated; EKG: arrhythmias, specifically SVT/V-tach, Sinus bradycardia, AV block and IVCDs possible; however, the EKG may be normal.

- Arterial Line Values: CI <1.8 L/min, PCWP >18 mmHg, SBP <90, MAP <60, Increased CVP and PAP.

Treatment includes:

- Dobutamine IV to increase cardiac contractility
- Norepinephrine IV if SBP <70
- Morphine can be given for pain; while potential for hypotension, it will decrease SNS response and decrease HR and MVO_2
- Treat underlying cause (e.g., papillary rupture = valve replacement)
- Intra-aortic Balloon Pump (IABP): Increases cardiac blood flow
- Re-vascularization if secondary to acute MI (CABG or PCI)

OBSTRUCTIVE SHOCK

Obstructive shock occurs when the preload (diastolic filling of the RV) of the heart is obstructed in one or several ways. There can be obstruction to the great vessels of the heart (such as from pulmonary embolism), there can be excessive afterload because the flow of blood out of the heart is obstructed (resulting in decreased cardiac output), or there can be direct compression of the heart, which can occur when blood or air fills the pericardial sac with cardiac tamponade or tension pneumothorax. Other causes include aortic dissection, vena cava syndrome, systemic hypertension, and cardiac lesions. Obstructive shock is often categorized with cardiogenic shock because of their similarities. **Signs and symptoms** of obstructive shock may vary depending on the underlying cause but typically include:

- Decrease in oxygen saturation
- Hemodynamic instability with hypotension and tachycardia, muffled heart sounds
- Chest pain
- Neurological impairment (disorientation, confusion)
- Dyspnea
- Impaired peripheral circulation (cool extremities, pallor)
- Generalized pallor and cyanosis

Treatment depends on the cause and may include oxygen, pericardiocentesis, needle thoracostomy or chest tube, and fluid resuscitation.

NEUROGENIC SHOCK

Neurogenic shock is a type of distributive shock that occurs when injury to the CNS from trauma resulting in acute spinal cord injury (from both blunt and penetrating injuries), neurological diseases, drugs, or anesthesia, impairs the autonomic nervous system that controls the cardiovascular system. The degree of symptoms relates to the level of injury with injuries above T1 capable of causing disruption of the entire sympathetic nervous system and lower injuries causing various degrees of disruption. Even incomplete spinal cord injury can cause neurogenic shock.

Symptoms include:

- Hypotension and warm dry skin related to lack of vascular tone that results in hypothermia from loss of cutaneous heat
- Bradycardia (common but not universal)

Treatment includes:

- ABCDE (airway, breathing, circulation, disability evaluation, exposure)
- Rapid fluid administration with crystalloid to keep mean arterial pressure at 85-90 mmHg
- Placement of pulmonary artery catheter to monitor fluid overload
- Inotropic agents (dopamine, dobutamine) if fluids don't correct hypotension
- Atropine for persistent bradycardia

ANAPHYLACTIC SHOCK

Anaphylactic reaction or anaphylactic shock may present with a few symptoms or a wide range of potentially lethal effects.

Symptoms may recur after the initial treatment (biphasic anaphylaxis), so careful monitoring is essential:

- Sudden onset of weakness, dizziness, confusion
- Severe generalized edema and angioedema; lips and tongue may swell
- Urticaria
- Increased permeability of vascular system and loss of vascular tone leading to severe hypotension and shock
- Laryngospasm/bronchospasm with obstruction of airway causing dyspnea and wheezing
- Nausea, vomiting, and diarrhea
- Seizures, coma, and death

Treatments:

- Establish patent airway and intubate if necessary, for ventilation
- Provide oxygen at 100% high flow
- Monitor VS
- Administer epinephrine (Epi-pen® or solution)
- Albuterol per nebulizer for bronchospasm
- Intravenous fluids to provide bolus of fluids for hypotension
- Diphenhydramine if shock persists
- Methylprednisolone if no response to other drugs

HYPOVOLEMIC SHOCK/VOLUME DEFICIT

Hypovolemic shock occurs when there is inadequate intravascular fluid. The loss may be *absolute* because of an internal shifting of fluid or an external loss of fluid, as occurs with massive hemorrhage, thermal injuries, severe vomiting or diarrhea, and internal injuries (such as ruptured spleen or dissecting arteries) that interfere with intravascular integrity. Hypovolemia may also be *relative* and related to vasodilation, increased capillary membrane permeability from sepsis or injuries, and decreased colloidal osmotic pressure that may occur with loss of sodium and some disorders, such as hypopituitarism and cirrhosis.

Hypovolemic shock is **classified** according to the degree of fluid loss:

- **Class I:** <750 mL or ≤15% of total circulating volume (TCV)
- **Class II:** 750-1500 mL or 15-30% of TCV
- **Class III:** 1500-2000 mL or 30-40% of TCV
- **Class IV:** >2000 mL or >40% of TCV

SYMPTOMS AND TREATMENT

Hypovolemic shock occurs when the total circulating volume of fluid decreases, leading to a fall in venous return that in turn causes a decrease in ventricular filling and preload, indicated by ↓ in right atrial pressure (RAP) and pulmonary artery occlusion pressure (PAOP). This results in a decrease in stroke volume and cardiac output. This in turn causes generalized arterial vasoconstriction, increasing afterload (↑ systemic vascular resistance), causing decreased tissue perfusion.

Symptoms: Anxiety, pallor, cool and clammy skin, delayed capillary refill, cyanosis, hypotension, increasing respirations, weak, thready pulse.

Treatment is aimed at identifying and treating the cause:

- Administration of blood, blood products, autotransfusion, colloids (such as plasma protein fraction), and/or crystalloids (such as normal saline)
- Oxygen; intubation and ventilation may be necessary
- Medications may include vasopressors, such as dopamine. NOTE: Fluids must be given before starting vasopressors!

NON-CARDIAC CHEST PAIN

Non-cardiac chest pain is pain that is similar in presentation to angina (pressure or severe pain in the chest that may extend to the neck, arms [especially left] and back) but is unrelated to coronary heart disease. Causes include:

- **Gastroesophageal reflux disease (GERD):** The most common cause of noncardiac pain. This pain is often relieved by drinking liquid and burping or taking antacids.
- **Bone/muscle disorders** of the chest, such as fibromyositis.
- **Esophageal abnormalities/disorders:** Contractions may cause painful spasms, or contractility may be weak/absent, allowing food to build up in the esophagus rather than moving into the stomach.
- **Pleuritis:** Inflammation of the pleura may result in sharp pain, generally on one side.
- **Gall bladder disease:** Referred pain from the gall bladder may occur in the midscapular, back, or right shoulder area.
- **Gastric ulcers**
- **Emotional stress, anxiety, panic attacks:** Patients often believe a panic attack is a heart attack, and fear then exacerbates the pain.

Behavioral and Psychosocial

SUBSTANCE ABUSE

Substance abuse is the abuse of drugs, medicines, or alcohol that causes mental and physical problems for the abuser and family. Abusers use substances out of boredom, to hide negative self-esteem, to dampen emotional pain, and to cope with daily stress. As the abuse continues, abusers become unable to take care of daily needs and duties. They lack effective coping mechanisms and the ability to make healthy choices. They can't identify and prioritize stress or choose positive behavior to resolve the stress in a healthy way. Some family members may act as codependents because of their desire to feel needed by the abuser, to control the person, and to stay with him or her. The nurse can help the family to confront an individual with their concerns about the person and their proposals for treatment. Family members can enforce consequences if treatment is not sought. Family members may also need counseling to learn new behaviors to stop enabling the abuser to continue substance abuse.

PATHOPHYSIOLOGY OF ADDICTION

Genetic, social, and personality factors may all play a role in the development of **addictive tendencies**. However, the main factor of the development of substance addiction is the pharmacological activation of the **reward system** located in the central nervous system (CNS). This reward systems pathway involves **dopaminergic neurons**. Dopamine is found in the CNS and is one of many neurotransmitters that play a role in an individual's mood. The mesolimbic pathway seems to play a primary role in the reward and motivational process involved with addiction. This pathway begins in the ventral tegmental area of the brain (VTA) and then moves forward into the nucleus accumbens located in the middle forebrain bundle (MFB). Some drugs enhance mesolimbic dopamine activity, therefore producing very potent effects on mood and behavior.

INDICATORS OF SUBSTANCE ABUSE

Many people with substance abuse (alcohol or drugs) are reluctant to disclose this information, but there are a number of **indicators** that are suggestive of substance abuse:

Physical signs:

- Burns on fingers or lips
- Pupils abnormally dilated or constricted, eyes watery
- Slurring of speech, slow speech
- Lack of coordination, instability of gait, tremors
- Sniffing repeatedly, nasal irritation, persistent cough
- Weight loss
- Dysrhythmias
- Pallor, puffiness of face
- Needle tracks on arms or legs
- Odor of alcohol/marijuana on clothing or breath

Behavioral signs:

- Labile emotions, including mood swings, agitation, and anger
- Inappropriate, impulsive, or risky behavior
- Lying
- Missing appointments
- Difficulty concentrating, short term memory loss, blackouts
- Insomnia or excessive sleeping; disoriented, confused
- Lack of personal hygiene

ALCOHOL WITHDRAWAL

Chronic abuse of ethanol (alcoholism) can lead to physical dependency. Sudden cessation of drinking, which often happens in the inpatient setting, is associated with **alcohol withdrawal syndrome.** It may be precipitated by trauma or infection and has a high mortality rate, 5-15% with treatment and 35% without treatment.

Signs/Symptoms: Anxiety, tachycardia, headache, diaphoresis, progressing to severe agitation, hallucinations, auditory/tactile disturbances, and psychotic behavior (delirium tremens).

Diagnosis: Physical assessment, blood alcohol levels (on admission).

Treatment includes:

- Medication: IV benzodiazepines to manage symptoms; electrolyte and nutritional replacement, especially magnesium and thiamine.
- Use the CIWA scale to measure symptoms of withdrawal; treat as indicated.
- Provide an environment with minimal sensory stimulus (lower lights, close blinds) & implement fall and seizure precautions.
- Prevention: Screen all patients for alcohol/substance abuse, using CAGE or other assessment tool. Remember to express support and comfort to patient; wait until withdrawal symptoms are subsiding to educate about alcohol use and moderation.

Therapeutic Interventions

Cardiac Procedures

CARDIAC CATHETERIZATION AND PERCUTANEOUS CORONARY INTERVENTION

A percutaneous coronary intervention (PCI) is indicated to treat symptoms of coronary artery disease. It should be considered for patients who experience angina or ECG changes during a stress test. PCI may be indicated if medical management is unsuccessful in patients with chest pain, dyspnea, or heart failure. A cardiac catheterization should also be considered for investigational purposes, in cases of cardiomegaly, congestive heart failure, valvular heart disease, and in evaluation of the need for heart transplantation.

An emergent cardiac catheterization and PCI should be considered for patients showing signs and symptoms of ST elevation myocardial infarction.

LEFT VS. RIGHT-SIDED CARDIAC CATHETERIZATION

Cardiac catheterization is a minimally-invasive procedure in which a catheter is inserted into the femoral or radial artery and threaded into the right or left side of the heart in order to diagnose, treat, or monitor cardiac conditions. Cardiac catheterization is fluoroscopy-guided, and contrast dye is injected for angiography.

Cardiac catheterization	Right heart	Left heart
Indications	Identify abnormal blood flow. Monitor cardiac and pulmonary pressures. Diagnose/treat cardiac tamponade, valve disease, HF, pulmonary hypertension, shock, congenital heart defects, and cardiomyopathy. Monitor damage and treatment for MI. Evaluate CO, LV filling pressure, PAWP, and oxygen saturation. Biopsy heart transplants.	Evaluate heart function: left ventricular and outflow obstruction. Diagnose cardiac tumor, valve disease, congenital heart defects, coronary artery disease.
Risks	Pneumothorax, cardiac tamponade, infection, embolism, hypotension, rupture of pulmonary artery, air embolism, and dysrhythmias (VT).	MI, cardiac tamponade, pulmonary embolism, stroke, dysrhythmias, transient hypotension (associated with volume of contrast), shock congestive heart failure, chest pain, PVC, PAC, VT, or VF (rare), and unstable angina.

TESTS PRIOR TO CARDIAC CATHETERIZATION

Prior to cardiac catheterization, a complete physical examination and past medical history intake is obtained from the patient. An electrocardiogram and chest x-ray are performed. Relevant blood work should include: 1) a complete blood count to rule out a low hemoglobin level, indicating reduced oxygen-carrying capacity, or a low platelet count, which would indicate an increased risk for bleeding; and, 2) a complete metabolic panel should be obtained to check for electrolyte imbalances. Except in cases of emergency, therapy for any electrolyte imbalances should be initiated prior to cardiac catheterization. Female patients should also receive a pregnancy test prior to cardiac catheterization, as x-rays are harmful to fetal development.

NURSING CONSIDERATIONS

Prior to the procedure, the patient and family should be informed of the purpose of the cardiac catheterization and the risks and benefits involved. The patient should be informed about what to expect during the procedure itself. It is also important to ascertain if the patient has any known allergies to contrast dye, strawberries, or shellfish, as allergies to these items will require pre-procedural medication with antihistamines and corticosteroids to prevent a reaction to the contrast dye used during the cardiac catheterization.

The patient should be NPO (fasting) for 4-6 hours prior to the procedure. Subcutaneous insulin dosages should be adjusted to take into account the patient's NPO status. Oral hypoglycemic agents such as metformin should be held for 24 to 48 hours prior to and after a cardiac catheterization as it may have nephrotoxic effects in conjunction with the contrast dye. Anticoagulation therapy should be held for 48 to 72 hours prior to the procedure to decrease risk of bleeding.

PROCEDURE

The patient is brought to the cardiac catheterization lab and placed on continuous cardiac monitoring. The area over the femoral artery is clipped and cleansed with alcohol. The area over the femoral artery is then numbed using a local anesthetic. The femoral artery is accessed using an introducer needle, and a sheath is slid over the needle to provide continuous access into the artery. A guide-wire is then inserted into the sheath, and threaded up the artery and into the heart. Using contrast dye and real-time x-ray imaging, the coronary arteries are explored for evidence of any occlusions. If an occlusion is located, an angioplasty balloon is slid over the guide wire, and guided to the occlusion site. In cases of balloon angioplasty, a balloon is inflated, pushing the atherosclerotic plaque aside and opening up the coronary artery to reperfuse the area. If necessary, a stent may be placed over the lesion to prevent reocclusion of the artery. In cases of PCI atherectomy procedures, catheter-introduced cutting devices are used to trim, suction, and remove the identified plaque deposits.

ELEVATED ACTIVATED CLOTTING TIME

Activated clotting time (ACT) measures the amount of time it takes for platelets to aggregate. Prior to a cardiac catheterization, the patient is given a bolus of heparin – typically 100 to 150 units/kg in order to elevate the patient's ACT. This is done to prevent clots from forming on the sheath or within the coronary artery. The patient's ACT is checked every 5 to 10 minutes during the cardiac catheterization, and additional heparin boluses may be administered to maintain an ACT level greater than 300 seconds.

Because the patient's clotting time remains elevated immediately after the procedure, some doctors prefer to wait until the patient's ACT normalizes before removing the femoral artery sheath. The sheath is may be left in the femoral artery, with the patient on strict bed rest, until their ACT is between 75 and 90 seconds.

CARDIAC CATHETERIZATION CLOSURE DEVICES

After the femoral artery sheath is removed, manual pressure may be applied to achieve hemostasis at the insertion site. Other noninvasive methods to apply necessary pressure on the site include the FemoStop or a C-clamp. While the pressure device is in place, the patient will be required to stay on

81

strict bed rest. Bed rest may continue for up to 12 hours after hemostasis has been achieved, depending on facility policy and the patient's risk factors for bleeding.

Invasive closure devices are typically placed by the physician based upon individual preference. Angio-Seal and VasoSeal are collagen plug devices that are inserted into the femoral artery to prevent bleeding. A Perclose is a suture that is placed directly into the artery to prevent bleeding. A SyvekPatch is a dressing that is placed over the insertion site to encourage hemostasis. The period of bed rest required with each of these closure devices is dependent upon specific manufacturer guidelines, but is typically less than that of compression devices.

Symptoms Experienced During Catheterization

The patient may experience a pinching and burning sensation at the insertion site of the local anesthetic. The patient may also experience a "flushing" sensation as the contrast dye is injected into the coronary arteries. There is a risk for nausea, vomiting, and cardiac palpitations as a result of injection of the contrast dye. Further, because they must lie still for an extended period of time, some patients may complain of back pain or stiffness. Patients with chronic back pain may be particularly susceptible to this discomfort. The patient may also have a brief moment of chest pain while the angioplasty balloon is inflated. After the balloon is deflated, a brief episode of cardiac dysrhythmias may occur as a result of the restoration of blood flow to ischemic cardiac tissues.

Intervention Complications

The most common risk involved in cardiac catheterization is bleeding at the catheter insertion site. This is partly due to the anticoagulation medications that are given during cardiac catheterization. The patient may also experience bruising or development of a hematoma at the insertion site. There is also a risk for an allergic reaction to the contrast dye. As a result of exposure to contrast dye, the patient is also at risk for subsequent kidney injury.

Though rare, perforation of the arterial wall can occur during the cardiac catheterization. The patient is also at risk for retroperitoneal bleed, and hypovolemia or hypotension. The most serious complications related to a cardiac catheterization are stroke as a result of a dislodged embolus, myocardial infarction, aortic dissection, or death.

Nursing Considerations

After a cardiac catheterization, the patient should stay on strict bed rest for a minimum of one hour, and potentially longer depending upon the type of closure device used. During that time, the patient should be closely monitored for bleeding, hematoma development, or the presence of a bruit at the sheath insertion site. Vital signs should be carefully monitored -- typically every 15 minutes for an hour, every 30 minutes for 2 hours, and then every hour for 4 hours. The patient can resume activity as tolerated within six hours after the PCI. The patient should be orally hydrated to help flush the contrast dye from their blood stream.

After the cardiac catheterization, the patient's BUN and creatinine should be checked to monitor for renal injury as a result of the contrast dye. A complete blood count should be obtained immediately after the procedure and again six hours afterward to monitor for any signs of bleeding. Any complaints of flank or lower back pain should be promptly investigated, as they may result from a retroperitoneal bleed.

Medications Used in Conjunction With Cardiac Catheterization

To decrease the risk of clot formation at the insertion site or within the stent, the patient is typically started on an antiplatelet agent to prevent platelet aggregation. The most common medication used for this purpose is a glycoprotein IIb/IIIa inhibitor such as eptifibatide. The patient will also receive unfractionated heparin to elevate the activated clotting time (ACT) and prevent platelet aggregation during the cardiac catheterization. Antiplatelet medications such as aspirin and clopidogrel are typically prescribed after the cardiac catheterization to prevent platelet aggregation on and around the stent.

Nitrates are given prior to cardiac catheterization to prevent angina, and after the procedure to treat chest pain related to vasospasm. Beta-blockers and ACE inhibitors may be prescribed after a myocardial infarction to decrease cardiac workload by lowering the heart rate and blood pressure. Ongoing lipid lowering agents may be prescribed to decrease the buildup of atherosclerotic plaque over time.

PERCUTANEOUS CORONARY INTERVENTION

Percutaneous coronary intervention (PCI) (AKA angioplasty with stent) is a minimally-invasive procedure in which a stent is placed in a coronary artery to improve blood flow in arteries blocked by atherosclerotic plaques. Indications include acute STEMI, non-ST-elevation ACS, angina (stable or unstable), or abnormal stress test findings. Contraindications include long-term treatment with antiplatelet medications and severe life-threatening comorbidities. A relative contraindication is coronary arteries of less than 1.5 mm diameter. **Procedure**:

- The patient must be NPO for at least 6 hours prior to procedure (unless the situation is emergent) and may have medications adjusted prior to procedure.
- The patient is positioned supine on table, an IV started, and cardiac monitoring initiated
- The patient is prepped and draped.
- The patient is administered conscious sedation and local anesthetic to insertion site (usually femoral or radial).
- The catheter is inserted and threaded to the heart and coronary arteries, contrast dye injected, images taken.
- The balloon catheter is positioned at the occluded area and balloon inflated and deflated a number of times.
- The stent is positioned and expanded to provide an open lumen for blood flow.
- The catheter is removed and pressure is applied to insertion site.
- The patient is monitored for complications, which can include MI, stroke, pulmonary embolism, and myocardial ischemia from distal embolus.

PERICARDIOCENTESIS

Pericardiocentesis is done with ultrasound guidance to diagnose pericardial effusion or with ECG and ultrasound guidance to relieve cardiac tamponade. **Pericardiocentesis** may be done as treatment for cardiac arrest or with presentation of PEA with increased jugular venous pressure. Non-hemorrhagic tamponade may be relieved in 60-90% of cases, but hemorrhagic tamponade requires thoracotomy, as blood will continue to accumulate until the cause of the hemorrhage is corrected. Resuscitation equipment must be available, including a defibrillator, intravenous line in place, and cardiac monitoring.

The **procedure** is as follows:

- Elevate the chest 45° to bring the heart closer to the chest wall, pre-medicate with atropine, and insert a nasogastric tube if indicated.
- Cleanse the skin with chlorhexidine or another appropriate cleanser.
- After insertion of the needle using ultrasound guidance, remove the obturator and attach a syringe for aspiration.
- The needle can often be replaced with a catheter after removal for drainage.
- A post-procedure chest x-ray should be done to check for pneumothorax.

Possible complications: Pneumo/hemothorax, coronary artery rupture, hepatic injury, dysrhythmias, and false negative/positive aspiration.

IABP

The **intra-aortic balloon pump (IABP)** is a catheter with an inflatable balloon at the tip, which is inserted through the femoral artery and threaded into the descending thoracic aorta. The balloon inflates during diastole to increase circulation to the coronary arteries and then deflates during systole to decrease afterload. It is indicated in patients experiencing cardiogenic/septic shock, acute heart failure, unstable angina, and papillary or ventricular septal rupture.

Contraindications: Aortic valve stenosis and large aortic aneurysms.

Complications: Stroke, peripheral ischemia, renal injury, air embolus, and arrhythmias.

Nursing considerations are as follows:

- **Placement:**
  - Too high: occludes the left subclavian artery, which results in dizziness and decreased radial pulse.
  - Too low: occludes the renal artery, which results in flank pain and a sudden decrease in urine output.
  - Preventing displacement: the patient cannot bend his or her knees, sit up, or flex the hips more than 45°. Patient should remain in a supine position.
- **Timing**: In ECG mode, the balloon should inflate in the T-wave and deflate with the R. Do site checks, I&O, neuro-checks, and vascular checks every hour.
- If a **gas-leak alarm sounds** OR **blood is visible in the catheter**, this indicates balloon rupture/damage to the catheter. Immediately shut down the machine, place the patient in the Trendelenburg position, and notify the physician.
- **Weaning**: Decrease balloon volume/frequency to wean. Use the flutter function to prevent embolus while the catheter is still in place. After removal, the physician will allow bleeding for five seconds to eject clots.

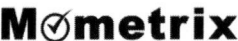

LEFT VENTRICULAR ASSIST DEVICE (LVAD)

The **left ventricular assist device** (LVAD) is implanted in the chest and takes blood from the base of the left ventricle though a cannula to the small LVAD pump and through an outflow cannula directly into the aorta to allow the left ventricle to rest. The LVAD pump is attached through a percutaneous line to an external controller and battery pack with rechargeable batteries. The LVAD is most commonly used for individuals with end-stage heart failure who are awaiting a heart transplant or as a destination treatment for those not candidates for transplantation. Individuals are sometimes able to stay on the LVAD for years with relief of many of their symptoms because the blood is circulating more effectively. A newer left ventricular assist device, the Impella 2.5, is an FDA-approved mini heart pump that is placed in the left ventricle through a catheter and activated by an external console. This device is used for temporary left ventricular assist during procedures, such as stenting or angioplasty.

Vascular Interventions

INDICATIONS FOR VASCULAR INTERVENTIONS

Vascular interventions are required when a patient has a condition that is decreasing blood flow to the limbs, causing ischemia-related damage. Conditions that require a vascular intervention include acute occlusion (embolus), severe unresponsive vascular disease, ruptured/dissecting aneurysm, damaged vessels, or congenital defect.

- **Bypass grafts:** The MD uses a harvested vein from another part of the body (saphenous usually) or synthetic graft to bypass the occlusion. Because veins have valves, they must be reversed or stripped of valves prior to attachment; however, synthetic grafts have a higher failure rate. A common peripheral bypass is the femoropopliteal (Fem-pop) bypass, extending from the femoral artery around the blockage to the popliteal artery.
- **Embolectomy:** A catheter is inserted into the blocked artery and threaded through the thrombus. Then a balloon on the tip is inflated, and the physician removes the catheter, removing the clot with it.
- **Aortic aneurysm repair:** This is an intense procedure, requiring an open incision and the patient to be placed on cardiopulmonary bypass. The affected area is resected and replaced with a vascular or Dacron graft.

Nursing considerations: Monitor and control blood pressure carefully to protect the patency and integrity of the grafts. Neurologic and renal function should also be carefully monitored, as emboli could block the renal or cerebral artery. Frequent neuro, urine output, vascular, and dressing checks.

Possible Complications: Pulmonary infection, graft-site infection, renal dysfunction, occlusion, hemorrhage, and embolus/thrombus.

PERIPHERAL ANGIOGRAPHY AND THE STENTING PROCEDURE

Peripheral angiography is a form of imaging to evaluate peripheral circulation and identify areas of blockage or abnormalities in the arteries of the lower extremities or (in rare occasions) the upper extremities. The procedure involves insertion of a catheter into the femoral artery (most common) or the radial or brachial artery and injection of iodine-based contrast medium to outline the arteries for imaging. Indications for peripheral angiography include peripheral arterial disease (claudication, ischemia) or peripheral arterial trauma. Prior to the procedure, patients may be advised to hold antithrombotic medications (such as anticoagulants) for a few days. The procedure is similar to that for PCI and cardiac catheterization and is usually carried out under conscious sedation and local anesthetic. If obstruction is noted per angiography, balloon angioplasty may be carried out and one or more wire coils or stents placed to maintain patency of the arteries and improve blood flow. Following the procedure, pressure is applied to the insertion site to prevent bleeding and the patient is monitored carefully for complications to the procedure, which may include stroke, MI, hemorrhage, vascular trauma, and impaired circulation of extremity.

ENDOVASCULAR GRAFTS

INDICATIONS

Endovascular grafting (AKA endovascular stent grafts or endovascular aneurysm repair [EVAR]) is a minimally-invasive procedure primarily used to treat thoracic or abdominal aortic aneurysms but can also be used on other aneurysms. During the procedure, an expandable stent graft (a fabric tube with wire mesh supports) attached to a catheter is inserted into the aorta, positioned at the aneurysm, and expanded to provide a secure open vessel and then the catheter removed. The graft extends both above and below the aneurysm to ensure blood flows only through the stent graft. Indications include:

- Aneurysm ≥5 cm in diameter.
- Dissecting aneurysm in risk of rupture.
- Rapidly growing aneurysm (greater than 1 cm/yr).
- Aneurysm with symptoms, such as severe pain, or chronic pain in back or abdomen.

Some patients are not candidates for endovascular graft because of the location of condition of the artery or preexisting conditions, such as Marfan disease.

PROCEDURE

The endovascular graft procedure is as follows:

- The patient generally stops taking anticoagulants, ASA, or NSAIDS a few days prior to the procedure.
- The patient is placed in supine position, prepped and draped, IV inserted, and cardiac monitoring carried out.
- Anesthesia varies but may include local with conscious sedation, general anesthesia, or spinal anesthesia.
- A spinal drainage catheter may be placed.
- Both right and left femoral arteries may be cannulated, contrast dye injected, and images taken to ensure accurate placement of catheters, and arch arteriogram for thoracic repair.
- The catheter with the graft is threaded to the aneurysm, positioned under fluoroscopy, and the stent released so that it expands above and below the aneurysm to prevent blood flow around the graft. In some cases, more than one graft is necessary.
- The catheter is removed and compression applied to insertion sites to prevent bleeding.

Complications include paralysis, infection, bleeding about the graft (endoleak), migration of the stent, kidney damage, and arterial occlusion. In some cases, a delayed rupture may still occur with endoleak.

CATHETER-DIRECTED THROMBOLYSIS

INDICATIONS

Catheter-directed thrombolysis is a minimally-invasive procedure used to dissolve thrombi by feeding a catheter through the common femoral artery to the site of occlusion and administration of a thrombolytic agent directly into the thrombus in order to improve blood flow and reduce symptoms. Fluoroscopy and a video monitor are used to ensure proper placement of the catheter and thrombolytic agent. Indications for catheter-directed thrombolysis include: acute ischemia of a limb, thrombosis associated with severe atherosclerosis, DVT, clotted dialysis fistula/graft, portal vein thrombosis, pulmonary embolus, and other emboli. Absolute contraindications to catheter-directed thrombolysis include: TIA or stroke within the previous 2 months, active bleeding or recent GI bleeding, history of neurological surgery, or intracranial trauma in the previous 3 months. Relative contraindications include a history of CPR or major surgery or trauma in the previous 10 days, hypertension >180/>110 mmHg, history of recent ophthalmic surgery, and intracranial tumor.

PROCEDURE

The catheter-directed thrombolysis procedure is as follows:

- The patient stops taking anticoagulants, ASA, or NSAIDS a few days prior to the procedure.
- The patient is NPO for at least 6 hours prior to the procedure.
- The patient is placed in supine position on the table and connected to a cardiac monitor.
- An IV line inserted to provide conscious sedation (or general anesthesia administered).
- The skin at insertion site (usually the femoral artery) is prepped, patient draped, and local anesthetic administered.
- The catheter inserted and contrast dye injected and images taken to ensure accurate placement of the catheter.
- Thrombolytic agent injected into the clot or a mechanical device used to break up the thrombus or suction it from the vessel.
- The catheter may be left in place for a few hours to 2 to 3 days and attached to a pump that delivers the thrombolytic agent at a specific rate until the clot dissolves.
- After catheter removal, compression applied to the site to prevent bleeding and the patient carefully monitored for complications, such as retroperitoneal hemorrhage, stroke, intracranial hemorrhage, or infection.

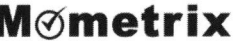

Cardiovascular Pharmacology

ANTIDYSRHYTHMICS

Antidysrhythmic drugs include a number of drugs that act on the conduction system, the ventricles and/or the atria to control dysrhythmias. There are four classes of drugs that are used as well as some that are unclassified:

- **Class I**: 3 subtypes of sodium channel blockers (quinidine, lidocaine, procainamide)
- **Class II**: β-receptor blockers (esmolol, propranolol)
- **Class III**: Slows repolarization (amiodarone, ibutilide)   ·
- **Class IV**: Calcium channel blockers (diltiazem, verapamil)
- **Unclassified**: Miscellaneous drugs with proven efficacy in controlling arrhythmias (adenosine, electrolyte supplements)

DIURETICS

Diuretics increase **renal perfusion and filtration**, thereby reducing preload and decreasing peripheral and pulmonary edema, hypertension, CHF, diabetes insipidus, and osteoporosis. There are different types of diuretics: loop, thiazide, and potassium sparing.

LOOP DIURETICS

Loop diuretics inhibit the reabsorption of sodium and chloride (primarily) in the ascending loop of Henle. They also cause increased secretion of other electrolytes, such as calcium, magnesium, and potassium, and this can result in imbalances that cause dysrhythmias. Other side effects include frequent urination, postural hypotension, and increased blood sugar and uric acid levels. They are short-acting so are less effective than other diuretics for control of hypertension.

- **Bumetanide** (Bumex®) is given intravenously after surgery to reduce preload or orally to treat heart failure.
- **Ethacrynic acid** (Edecrin®) is given intravenously after surgery to reduce preload.
- **Furosemide** (Lasix®) is used for the control of congestive heart failure as well as renal insufficiency. It is used after surgery to decrease preload and to reduce the inflammatory response caused by cardiopulmonary bypass (post-perfusion syndrome).

> **Review Video: Diuretics**
> Visit mometrix.com/academy and enter code: 373276

THIAZIDE DIURETICS

Thiazide diuretics inhibit the **reabsorption of sodium and chloride** primarily in the early distal tubules, forcing more sodium and water to be excreted. Thiazide diuretics increase secretion of potassium and bicarbonate, so they are often given with supplementary potassium or in combination with potassium-sparing diuretics. Thiazide diuretics are the first line of drugs for treatment of **hypertension**. They have a long duration of action (12-72 hours, depending on the drug) so they are able to maintain control of hypertension better than short-acting drugs. They may be given daily or 3–5 days per week. There are numerous thiazide diuretics, including:

- Chlorothiazide (Diuril®)
- Bendroflumethiazide (Naturetin®)
- Chlorthalidone (Hygroton®)
- Trichlormethiazide (Naqua®)

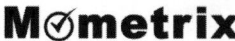

Side effects include, dizziness, lightheadedness, postural hypotension, headache, blurred vision, and itching, especially during initial treatment. Thiazide diuretics cause sensitivity to sun exposure, so people should be counseled to use sunscreen.

POTASSIUM-SPARING DIURETICS

Potassium-sparing diuretics inhibit the **reabsorption of sodium** in the late distal tubule and collecting duct. They are weaker than thiazide or loop diuretics, but do not cause a reduction in potassium level; however, if used alone, they may cause an increase in potassium, which can cause weakness, irregular pulse, and cardiac arrest. Because potassium-sparing diuretics are less effective alone, they are often given in a combined form with a thiazide diuretic (usually chlorothiazide), which mitigates the potassium imbalance. Typical side effects include dehydration, blurred vision, nausea, insomnia, and nasal congestion, especially in the first few days of treatment.

- **Spironolactone** (Aldactone®) is a synthetic steroid diuretic that increases the secretion of both water and sodium and is used to treat congestive heart failure. It may be given orally or intravenously.
- **Eplerenone** is an antimineralocorticoid similar to spironolactone but with fewer side effects.

SMOOTH MUSCLE RELAXANTS

Smooth muscle relaxants decrease peripheral vascular resistance, but may cause hypotension and headaches.

- Sodium nitroprusside (Nipride®) dilates both arteries and veins; rapid-acting and used for reduction of hypertension and afterload reduction for heart failure.
- Nitroglycerin (Tridil®) primarily dilates veins and is used sublingual or IV to reduce preload for acute heart failure, unstable angina, and acute MI. Nitroglycerin may also be used prophylactically after PCIs to prevent vasospasm.
- Hydralazine (Apresoline®) dilates arteries and is given intermittently to reduce hypertension.

CALCIUM CHANNEL BLOCKERS

Calcium channel blockers are primarily arterial vasodilators that may affect the peripheral and/or coronary arteries.

- Side effects: Lethargy, flushing, edema, ascites, and indigestion:
- Nifedipine (Procardia®) and nicardipine (Cardene®) are primarily arterial vasodilators, used to treat acute hypertension. Diltiazem (Cardizem®) and Verapamil (Calan®, Isoptin®) dilate primarily coronary arteries and slow the heart rate, thus are used for angina, atrial fibrillation, and SVT. *Note:* Nifedipine (Procardia®) should be avoided in older adults due to increased risk of hypotension and myocardial ischemia.

> **Review Video: Calcium Channel Blockers and Antiarrhythmics**
> Visit mometrix.com/academy and enter code: 942825

ADDITIONAL VASODILATORS

B-type natriuretic peptide (BNP) (Nesiritide [Natrecor®]) is type of vasodilator (non-inotropic), which is a recombinant form of a peptide of the human brain. It decreases filling pressure, vascular resistance, and increases U/O.

- May cause hypotension, headache, bradycardia, and nausea. It is used short term for worsening decompensated CHF; contraindicated in SBP<90, cardiogenic shock, constrictive pericarditis, or valve stenosis.

Alpha-adrenergic blockers block alpha receptors in arteries and veins, causing vasodilation.

- May cause orthostatic hypotension and edema from fluid retention.
- Labetalol (Normodyne®) is a combination peripheral alpha-blocker and cardiac β-blocker that is used to treat acute hypertension, acute stroke, and acute aortic dissection.
- Phentolamine (Regitine®) is a peripheral arterial dilator that reduces afterload. It is used for HTN crisis in patients with pheochromocytoma, as well as a subcutaneous injection for extravasation of vesicants.

Selective specific dopamine DA-1-receptor agonists:

- Fenoldopam (Corlopam®) is a peripheral dilator affecting renal and mesenteric arteries and can be used for patients with renal dysfunction or those at risk of renal insufficiency.

INOTROPIC AGENTS

Inotropic agents are drugs used to increase cardiac output and improve contractibility. IV inotropic agents may increase the risk of death, but may be used when other drugs fail. Oral forms of these drugs are less effective than intravenous. Inotropic agents include:

- **β-Adrenergic agonists:**
  - **Dobutamine** improves cardiac output, treats cardiac decompensation, and increases blood pressure. It helps the body to utilize norepinephrine. Side effects include increased or labile blood pressure, increased heart rate, PVCs, N/V, and bronchospasm.
  - **Dopamine** improves cardiac output, blood pressure, and blood flow to the renal and mesenteric arteries. Side effects include tachycardia or bradycardia, palpitations, BP changes, dyspnea, nausea and vomiting, headache, and gangrene of extremities.
- **Phosphodiesterase III inhibitors:**
  - **Milrinone** (Primacor®) increases strength of contractions and cause vasodilation. Side effects include ventricular arrhythmias, hypotension, and headaches.
- **Digoxin (Lanoxin®)** increases contractibility and cardiac output and prevents arrhythmias.

DIGOXIN

Digitalis drugs, most commonly administered in the form of digoxin (Lanoxin), are derived from the foxglove plant and are used to increase myocardial contractility, left ventricular output, and slow conduction through the AV node, decreasing rapid heart rates and promoting diuresis. Digoxin does not affect mortality, but increases tolerance to activity and reduces hospitalizations for heart failure. Therapeutic levels (0.5-2.0 ng/mL) should be maintained to avoid digitalis toxicity, which can occur even if digoxin levels are within therapeutic range, so observation of symptoms is critical. Because patients with heart failure are often on diuretics which decrease potassium levels, they are at increased risk for toxicity.

Symptoms of toxicity are as follows:

- Early signs: Increasing fatigue, lethargy, depression, and nausea and vomiting; progress to severe diarrhea, blurred vision/yellow or green halos around lights, fatigue/weakness
- Arrythmias: SA or AV block, VT/VF, PVCs, and bradycardia

Treatment consists of the following:

- Monitor serum levels and symptoms.
- Digoxin immune FAB (Digibind®) may be used to bind to digoxin and inactivate it if necessary.

GLYCOPROTEIN IIB/IIIA INHIBITORS

Glycoprotein IIB/IIIA Inhibitors are drugs that are used to inhibit platelet binding and prevent clots prior to and following invasive cardiac procedures, such as angioplasty and stent placement. These medications are used in combination with anticoagulant drugs, such as heparin and aspirin for the following:

- Acute coronary syndromes (ACS), such as unstable angina or myocardial infarctions
- Percutaneous coronary intervention (PCI), such as angioplasty and stent placement

These medications are contraindicated in those with a low platelet count or active bleeding:

- **Eptifibatide (Integrilin®):** Used with both heparin and aspirin for ACS and PCI and affects platelet binding for 6-8 hours after administration. Should not be used in patients with renal problems.
- **Tirofiban (Aggrastat®):** Used with heparin for PCI patients with reduced dosage for those with renal problems and affects platelet binding for only 4-8 hours after administration.

PHARMACOLOGIC MEASURES TO MAXIMIZE PERFUSION

The primary focus of pharmacologic measures to **maximize perfusion** is to reduce the risk of **thromboses**:

- **Antiplatelet agents**, such as aspirin, Ticlid®, and Plavix®, which interfere with the function of the plasma membrane, interfering with clotting. These agents are ineffective to treat clots but prevent clot formation.
- **Vasodilators** may divert blood from ischemic areas, but some may be indicated, such as Pletal®, which dilates arteries and decreases clotting, and is used for control of intermittent claudication.
- **Antilipemic**, such as Zocor® and Questran®, slow progression of atherosclerosis.
- **Hemorheologic agents**, such as Trental®, reduce fibrinogen, reducing blood viscosity and rigidity of erythrocytes; however, clinical studies show limited benefit. It may be used for intermittent claudication.
- **Analgesics** may be necessary to improve quality of life. Opioids may be needed in some cases.
- **Thrombolytics** may be injected into a blocked artery under angiography to dissolve clots.
- **Anticoagulants**, such as Coumadin® and Lovenox®, prevent blood clots from forming.

ADMINISTRATION OF FIBRINOLYTIC (THROMBOLYTIC) INFUSIONS FOR MI

Fibrinolytic infusion is indicated for acute myocardial infarction under these conditions:

- Symptoms of MI, <6-12 hours since onset of symptoms
- ≥1 mm elevation of ST in ≥2 contiguous leads
- No contraindications and no cardiogenic shock

Fibrinolytic agents should be administered as soon as possible, within 30 minutes is best. All agents convert plasminogen to plasmin, which breaks down fibrin, dissolving clots:

- Streptokinase and anistreplase (1st generation)
- Alteplase or tissue plasminogen activator (tPA) (2nd generation)
- Reteplase and tenecteplase (3rd generation)

Contraindications

- Present or recent bleeding or history of severe bleeding
- History of intracranial hemorrhage
- History of stroke (<3 months unless within 3 hours)
- Aortic dissection or pericarditis
- Intracranial/intraspinal surgery or trauma within 3 months or neoplasm, aneurysm, or AVM

Relative contraindications

- Active peptic ulcer
- >10 minutes of CPR
- Advanced renal or hepatic disease
- Pregnancy
- Anticoagulation therapy
- Acute uncontrolled hypertension or chronic poorly controlled hypertension
- Recent (2–4 weeks) internal bleeding
- Non-compressible vascular punctures

Electrophysiologic Interventions

PACEMAKERS

Pacemakers are used to stimulate the heart when the normal conduction system of the heart is defective. **Pacemakers** may be used temporarily or be permanently implanted. Temporary pacemakers for external cardiac pacing are commonly used in the emergency setting. Temporary pacemakers may be used prophylactically or therapeutically to treat a cardiac abnormality. Clinical uses include:

- To treat persistent **dysrhythmias** not responsive to medications
- To increase **cardiac output** with bradydysrhythmia by increasing rate
- To decrease **ventricular or supraventricular tachycardia** by "overdrive" stimulation of contractions
- To treat **secondary heart block** caused by myocardial infarction, ischemia, and drug toxicity
- To improve **cardiac output** after cardiac surgery
- To provide **diagnostic information** through electrophysiology studies, which induce dysrhythmias for purposes of evaluation
- To provide **pacing** when a permanent pacemaker malfunctions

> **Review Video: Pacemaker Care**
> Visit mometrix.com/academy and enter code: 979075

TRANSCUTANEOUS PACING

Transcutaneous pacing is used temporarily in an emergency situation to treat symptomatic bradydysrhythmias that don't respond to medications (atropine) and result in hemodynamic instability. Generally, the patient is provided oxygen and some sort of mild sedation before the pacing. The placement of pacing pads is usually one pacing pad (negative) on the left chest, inferior to the clavicle, and the other (positive) on the left back, inferior to the scapula, so the heart is sandwiched between the two. Lead wires attach the pads to the monitor. The rate of pacing is usually set around 80 bpm. The current is increased slowly until capture occurs—a spiking followed by QRS sequence—then the current is readjusted downward if possible just to maintain capture, keeping it 5-10 mA above the pacing threshold. Both demand and fixed modes are available, but demand mode is preferred. The patient should be warned that the shocks may induce pain.

EPICARDIAL PACING

Epicardial pacing wires may be attached directly to the exterior atria, ventricles, or both at the conclusion of surgery for CPB or valve repair in the event that postoperative pacing support is required or for those with risk of AV block because of medications used to control atrial fibrillation. Cold cardioplegia may precipitate the transient sinus node or AV node dysfunction. While some surgeons avoid placing epicardial pacing wires because of concerns about bleeding and cardiac tamponade on removal, recommendations include placing at least one ventricular pacing wire. A typical configuration for pacing wires is atrial pacing wires placed in a plastic disk that is sutured low on the right atrium. The two ventricular wires are attached over the right ventricular wall. Atrial pacing wires may be used to record atrial activity and, and with standard ECG, can help to distinguish atrial and junctional arrhythmias and ventricular arrhythmias. Pacing wires can also be used therapeutically to increase the heart rate to about 90 bpm in order to achieve optimal hemodynamics. The epicardial leads are intended for use of 7 days or less and may be less reliable if used for extended periods. The wires are removed by applying gentle traction.

TEMPORARY TRANSVENOUS PACEMAKERS

Transvenous pacemakers, comprised of a catheter with a lead at the end, may be used prophylactically or therapeutically on a temporary basis to treat symptomatic bradycardias or heart blocks when other methods have failed. The catheter has a balloon tip that must be checked for leaks prior to insertion – this is usually done by inflating the catheter tip while submersed in normal saline and checking for bubbles. After the balloon's integrity is verified, the catheter is inserted through the femoral or jugular vein and the balloon is inflated. The catheter is then attached to an external pulse generator, and the settings are adjusted to achieve capture. The balloon is then deflated, and placement can be verified via ultrasound or chest x-ray.

Complications are similar to those of PCI and permanent pacemaker insertion, including infection, hemorrhage, catheter migration, perforation, embolism, thrombosis, and pacemaker syndrome.

TRANSVENOUS PACER SETTINGS

Temporary transvenous pacing utilizes bipolar leads with two tails, positive/proximal and negative/distal, and these must be connected properly to the pulse generator, with the distal end of the pacing lead to the negative terminal and the proximal end to the positive terminal. Once the transvenous pacing wire is inserted and the leads are connected to the pulse generator, it must be set to the patient's needs:

- **Rate**: The beats per minute are usually set between 70 and 80 (allowable range is generally 50-90), but this may vary according to individual needs.
- **Sensitivity**: The myocardial voltage needed for the pacing electrode to detect P or R waves. The sensitivity is usually set at 2 mV and then adjusted as needed to ensure capture. Most pacemakers can sense 0.3-10.0 mV from the atria and 0.8-29.0 mV from the ventricles, but setting it relatively low prevents oversensing.
- **Output**: The current or pulse produced by the pulse generator is usually set at 5 mA. The current is delivered rapidly, in about 0.6 ms.

PROBLEMS RELATED TO TRANSVENOUS PACING

With transvenous pacing (usually per a pulse generator connected to a pacing cable and a pacing wire, which is inserted into the right internal jugular to the right ventricle for ventricular pacing and right atrium for atrial pacing), sensing refers to the ability to detect electrical activity of the heart. Capture occurs when an artificial stimulus (the pulse generator) depolarizes the heart, indicated by a pacer spike followed by the QRS complex.

Problems include:

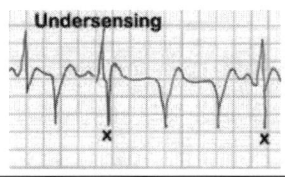	**Undersensing**: The sensitivity is too low to detect cardiac depolarizations, and triggers unneeded contractions, competing with the patient's native rhythm. This may be related to the dislodging of the lead, incorrect positioning of the lead, or a low-amplitude cardiac signal.
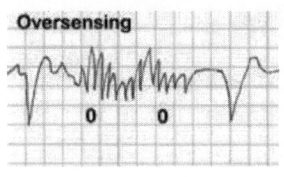	**Oversensing**: The sensitivity is too high and misinterprets artifacts (such as muscle contractions) and non-depolarization events as contractions and fails to trigger, resulting in decreased cardiac output because of the interruption in contractions. This may result from damage or disconnection of the lead.
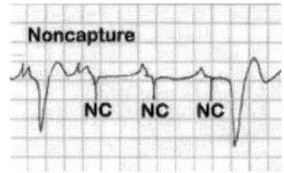	**Noncapture**: The pacemaker does not trigger contractions. This may be related to settings, lead disconnection, low battery, or metabolic changes.

PACEMAKER COMPLICATIONS

Pacemakers, transvenous and permanent, are invasive foreign bodies and, as such, can cause a number of different **complications**:

- Infection, bleeding, or hematoma may occur at the entry site of leads for temporary pacemakers or at the subcutaneous area of implantation for permanent generators.
- Puncture of the subclavian vein or internal mammary artery may cause a hemothorax.
- The endocardial electrode may irritate the ventricular wall, causing ectopic beats or tachycardia.
- Dislodgement of the transvenous lead may lead to malfunction or perforation of the myocardium. This is one of the most common early complications.
- Dislocation of leads may result in phrenic nerve or muscle stimulation (which may be evidenced by hiccupping).
- Cardiac tamponade may result when the epicardial wires of temporary pacing are removed.
- General malfunctioning of the pacemaker may indicate dislodgement, dislocation, interference caused by electromagnetic fields, and the need for new batteries or a new generator.
- Pacemaker syndrome

PACEMAKER SYNDROME

Pacemaker syndrome can occur with any type of pacemaker if there is inadequate synchronicity between the contractions of the atria and ventricles, resulting in a decrease in cardiac output and inadequate atrial contribution to the filling of the ventricles. Total peripheral vascular resistance may increase to maintain blood pressure, but hypotension occurs after decompensation.

- **Mild**
  - Pulsations evident in the neck and abdomen
  - Cardiac palpitations
  - Headache and feeling of anxiety
  - General malaise and unexplained weakness
  - Pain or feeling of fullness in jaw and/or chest
- **Moderate**
  - Increasing dyspnea on exertion with accompanying orthopnea
  - Dizziness, vertigo, and increasing confusion
  - Feeling of choking
- **Severe**
  - Increasing pulmonary edema with dyspnea even at rest
  - Crackling rales
  - Syncope
  - Heart failure

AUTOMATIC ICD

The **automatic implantable cardioverter-defibrillator (AICD)** is similar to the pacemaker and is implanted in the same way, with one or more leads to the ventricular myocardium or the epicardium, but it is used to control tachycardia and/or fibrillation. Most AICDs consist of a pacing/sensing electrode, a pulse generator, and defibrillation electrodes. Severe tachycardia may be related to electrical disturbances, cardiomyopathy, or postoperative response to the repair of congenital disease. In some cases, it is not responsive to medications. When the pulse reaches a certain preset rate, then the device automatically provides a small electrical impulse to the atrial or ventricular myocardium to slow the heart. If fibrillation occurs, a higher energy shock is delivered. It takes 5-15 seconds for the device to detect abnormalities in the pulse rate, and more than one shock may be required so fainting can occur. Contemporary devices can function as both a pacemaker and an ICD, which is especially important for those who have episodes of both bradycardia and tachycardia. The use of adjunctive antiarrhythmics or ablation is important to prevent AICD shocks.

WEARABLE CARDIOVERTER DEFIBRILLATOR

A wearable cardioverter defibrillator (such as a LifeVest) is a non-invasive defibrillator that operates automatically and does not require the assistance of a second person. The LifeVest is used to prevent sudden cardiac death (SCD) in patients who are increased risk. It may be used temporarily while awaiting implantation of an ICD or for prolonged periods if not a candidate. Indications include heart failure with EF <35%, survival of previous cardiac arrest related to VT/VF, and arrhythmias post MI. Patients who are in the 3-month waiting period while attempting other therapy, <40 days post MI, awaiting heart transplantation, or have life expectancy of <1 year are candidates for the wearable cardioverter defibrillator. The vest has electrodes to monitor heart function and treatment pads to deliver shocks. The vest is placed next to the skin and secured snugly. A gong alarm alerts the patient that some problem is occurring, such as too loose vest. If the device detects a shockable rhythm, the vibration alert occurs, followed by siren alert, and voice prompts. The patient can press the response buttons to stop the shock. The shocking electrodes automatically release conductive gel and a treatment shock occurs.

CARDIAC ABLATION PROCEDURE

The cardiac ablation procedure includes the following:

- **Pretesting**: Blood tests (may vary) and ECG is carried out.
- All usual heart and blood pressure medications are usually taken in the morning before the procedure unless otherwise advised by physician.
- The patient should ingest only water the morning of the test and no fluids for 3 to 6 hours before test.
- An IV line is placed in the arm for administration of anesthetic agent and fluids and ECG monitoring electrodes applied.
- The patient is transported to the electrophysiology laboratory, placed on the table, and draped. For A-fib, defibrillation pads are applied to the patient's back.
- Conscious sedation is administered. Heavier sedation is usually needed for A-fib ablation.
- Local anesthetic is applied to catheter insertion sites (commonly femoral artery or vein). For long procedures, a urinary catheter is inserted.
- Three catheters (intracardiac ultrasound for viewing, ablation catheter, and mapping catheter to detect electrical activity) are inserted and advanced into the heart. For A-fib ablation, 5 catheters are inserted, 3 in one femoral vein or artery and 2 in the other.
- Ablation procedures are carried out using heat (radiofrequency) and/or cold (cryotherapy) to scar the tissue, interfering with transmission of impulses.
- Catheters are removed, compression applied to prevent bleeding, and patient monitored for complications.

INDICATIONS AND POST-OPERATIVE CARE

Cardiac ablation is a minimally invasive procedure to treat atrial fibrillation and SVT uncontrolled by medications. Cardiac ablation is used for cardiac rhythm disorders (supraventricular tachycardia/arrhythmias) arising from the atria, including AV nodal reentry tachycardia (AVNRT), atrioventricular reentrant tachycardia (AVRT), atrial tachycardia (AT), and atrial flutter (AFL) as well as atrial fibrillation (A-fib). A-fib ablation (pulmonary vein isolation procedure) is more complex because the catheters must be positioned in the left atrium, and the procedure may need to be repeated more than once. Serious complications (such as hemorrhage, stroke, or MI) are rare.

Following the procedure, the patient is monitored in the recovery room. Once stable, the patient is returned to the room. The patient must remain in supine position with head elevated no more than 30 degrees for 4 to 6 hours and must be advised to avoid crossing the legs. A compression dressing or device is placed at the insertion site(s) to prevent bleeding, and the sites must be assessed frequently.

CARDIOVERSION

Cardioversion sends a timed electrical stimulation to the heart to convert a tachydysrhythmia (such as atrial fibrillation) to a normal sinus rhythm. Usually, anticoagulation therapy is done for at least 3 weeks prior to elective cardioversion to reduce the risk of emboli, and digoxin is discontinued for at least 48 hours prior. During the procedure, the patient is usually sedated and/or anesthetized. Electrodes in the form of gel-covered paddles or pads are placed in the anteroposterior position and then connected by leads to a computerized ECG and cardiac monitor with a defibrillator. The defibrillator is synchronized with the ECG so that the electrical current is delivered during ventricular depolarization (QRS). The timing must be precise in order to prevent ventricular tachycardia or ventricular fibrillation. Sometimes, drug therapy is used in conjunction with cardioversion; for example, antiarrhythmics (Cardizem®, Cordarone®) may be given before the procedure to slow the heart rate.

Arrhythmia	Beginning Monophasic Shock	Beginning Biphasic Shock
Atrial Fibrillation	50-100 J	25 J
Atrial Flutter	25-50 J	15 J
Ventricular Tachycardia	100-200 J	50 J

DEFIBRILLATION

Emergency defibrillation delivers a non-synchronized shock that is given to treat acute ventricular fibrillation, pulseless ventricular tachycardia, or polymorphic ventricular tachycardia with a rapid rate and decompensating hemodynamics. **Defibrillation** can be given at any point in the cardiac cycle. It causes depolarization of myocardial cells, which can then repolarize to regain a normal sinus rhythm. Defibrillation delivers an electrical discharge through pads/paddles. In an acute care setting, the preferred position to place the pads is the anteroposterior position. In this position, one pad is placed to the right of the sternum about the second to third intercostal space, and the other pad is placed between the left scapula and the spinal column. This decreases the chances of damaging implanted devices, such as pacemakers, and this positioning has also been shown to be more effective for external cardioversion (if indicated at some point during resuscitation). There are two main types of defibrillator shock waveforms: monophasic and biphasic. Biphasic defibrillators deliver a shock in one direction for half of the shock, and then in the return direction for the other half, making them more effective and able to be used at lower energy levels. Monophasic defibrillation is given at 200-360 J and biphasic defibrillation is given at 100-200 J.

Respiratory

NON-INVASIVE VENTILATION

NASAL CANNULA

A nasal cannula can be used to deliver supplemental oxygen to a patient, but it is only useful for flow rates ≤6 L/min as higher rates are drying of the nasal passages. As it is not an airtight system, some ambient air is breathed in as well so oxygen concentration ranges from about 24-44%. The nasal cannula does not allow for control of respiratory rate, so the patient must be able to breathe independently.

NON-REBREATHER MASK

A non-rebreather mask can be used to deliver higher concentrations (60-90%) of oxygen to those patients who are able to breathe independently. The mask fits over the nose and mouth and is secured by an elastic strap. A 1.5 L reservoir bag is attached and connects to an oxygen source. The bag is inflated to about 1 liter at a rate of 8-15 L/min before the mask is applied as the patient breathes from this reservoir. A one-way exhalation valve prevents most exhaled air from being rebreathed.

NON-INVASIVE POSITIVE PRESSURE VENTILATORS

Non-invasive positive pressure ventilators provide air through a tight-fitting nasal or face mask, usually pressure cycled, avoiding the need for intubation and reducing the danger of hospital-acquired infection and mortality rates. It can be used for acute respiratory failure and pulmonary edema. There are 2 types of non-invasive positive pressure ventilators:

- **CPAP (Continuous positive airway pressure)** provides a steady stream of pressurized air throughout both inspiration and expiration. CPAP improves breathing by decreasing preload for patients with congestive heart failure. It reduces the effort required for breathing by increasing residual volume and improving gas exchange.
- **Bi-PAP (Bi-level positive airway pressure)** provides a steady stream of pressurized air as CPAP but it senses inspiratory effort and increases pressure during inspiration. Bi-PAP pressures for inspiration and expiration can be set independently. Machines can be programmed with a backup rate to ensure a set number of respirations per minute.

NEVER place a patient in wrist restraints while wearing these devices. If the patient vomits, they need to be able to remove the mask to prevent aspiration.

FACE MASK

Ensuring that a face mask (Ambu bag) is the correct fit and type is important for adequate ventilation, oxygenation, and prevention of aspiration. Difficulties in management of face mask ventilation relate to risk factors: >55 years, obesity, beard, edentulous, and history of snoring. In some cases, if dentures are adhered well, they may be left in place during induction. The face mask is applied by lifting the mandible (jaw thrust) to the mask and avoiding pressure on soft tissue. Oral or nasal airways may be used, ensuring that the distal end is at the angle of the mandible. There are a number of steps to prevent mask airway leaks:

- Increasing or decreasing the amount of air to the mask to allow better seal
- Securing the mask with both hands while another person ventilates

- Accommodating a large nose by using the mask upside down
- Utilizing a laryngeal mask airway if excessive beard prevents seal

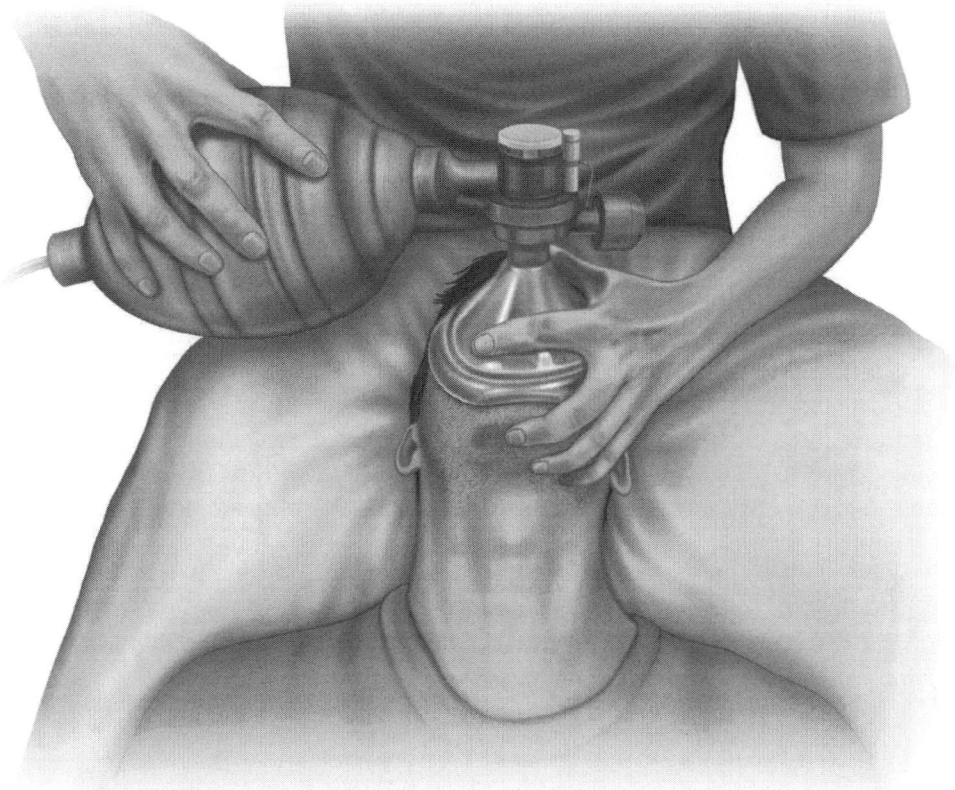

HIGH AND LOW FLOW OXYGEN DELIVERY

High flow oxygen delivery devices provide oxygen at flow rates higher than the patient's inspiratory flow rate at specific medium to high FiO₂, up to 100%. However, a flow of 100% oxygen actually provides only 60-80% FiO₂ to the patient because the patient also breathes in some room air, diluting the oxygen. The actual amount of oxygen received depends on the type of interface or mask. Additionally, the flow rate is actually less than the inspiratory flow rate upon actual delivery. High flow oxygen delivery is usually not used in the sleep center. Humidification is usually required because the high flow is drying.

Low flow oxygen delivery devices provide 100% oxygen at flow rates lower than the patient's inspiratory flow rate, but the oxygen mixes with room air, so the FiO₂ varies. Humidification is usually only required if flow rate is >3L/min. Much oxygen is wasted with exhalation, so a number of different devices to conserve oxygen are available. Interfaces include transtracheal catheters and cannulae with reservoirs.

AIRWAY DEVICES
OROPHARYNGEAL, NASOPHARYNGEAL, AND TRACHEOSTOMY TUBES

Airways are used to establish a patent airway and facilitate respirations:

- **Oropharyngeal**: This plastic airway curves over the tongue and creates space between the mouth and the posterior pharynx. It is used for anesthetized or unconscious patients to keep tongue and epiglottis from blocking the airway.

- **Nasopharyngeal** (trumpet): This smaller flexible airway is more commonly used in conscious patients and is inserted through one nostril, extending to the nasopharynx. It is commonly utilized in patients who need frequent suctioning.
- **Tracheostomy tubes**: Tracheostomy may be utilized for mechanical ventilation. Tubes are inserted into the opening in the trachea to provide a conduit and maintain the opening. The tube is secured with ties around the neck. Because the air entering the lungs through the tracheostomy bypasses the warming and moistening effects of the upper airway, air is humidified through a room humidifier or through the delivery of humidified air through a special mask or mechanical ventilation. If the tracheostomy is going to be long-term, eventually a stoma will form at the site, and the tube can be removed.

LARYNGEAL MASK AIRWAY

The laryngeal-mask airway (LMA) is an intermediate airway allowing ventilation but not complete respiratory control. The LMA consists of an inflatable cuff (the mask) with a connecting tube. It may be used temporarily before tracheal intubation or when tracheal intubation can't be done. It can also be a conduit for later blind insertion of an endotracheal tube. The head and neck must be in neutral position for insertion of the LMA. If the patient has a gag reflex, conscious sedation or topical anesthesia (deep oropharyngeal) is required. The LMA is inserted by sliding along the hard palate, using the finger as a guide, into the pharynx, and the ring is inflated to create a seal about the opening to the larynx, allowing ventilation with mild positive-pressure. The ProSeal® LMA has a modified cuff that extends onto the back of the mask to improve seal. LMA is contraindicated in morbid obesity, obstructions or abnormalities of oropharynx, and non-fasting patients, as some aspiration is possible even with the cuff seal inflated.

ESOPHAGEAL-TRACHEAL COMBITUBE®

The esophageal tracheal Combitube® (ETC) is an intermediate airway that contains two lumens and can be inserted into either the trachea or the esophagus (≤91%). The twin-lumen tube has a proximal cuff providing a seal of the oropharynx and a distal cuff providing a seal about the distal tube. Prior to insertion, the Combitube® cuffs should be checked for leaks (15 mL of air into distal and 85 mL of air into proximal). The patient should be non-responsive and with absent gag reflex with head in neutral position. The tube is passed along the tongue and into the pharynx, utilizing markings on the tube (black guidelines) to determine depth by aligning the ETC with the upper incisors or alveolar ridge. Once in place the distal cuff is inflated (10-15 mL) and then placement in the trachea or esophagus should be determined, so the proper lumen for ventilation can be used. The proximal cuff is inflated (usually to 50-75 mL) and ventilation begun. A capnogram should be used to confirm ventilation.

MECHANICAL VENTILATION
ENDOTRACHEAL INTUBATION

Endotracheal intubation is often necessary with respiratory failure for control of hypoxemia, hypercapnia, hypoventilation, and/or obstructed airway. Equipment should be assembled and tubes and connections checked for air leaks with a 10 mL syringe. The mouth and/or nose should be cleaned of secretions and suctioned if necessary. The patient should be supine with the patient's head level with the lower sternum of the clinician. With orotracheal/endotracheal intubation, the clinician holds the laryngoscope (in left hand) and inserts it into right corner of mouth, the epiglottis is lifted and the larynx exposed. A thin flexible intubation stylet may be used and the endotracheal tube (ETT) (in right hand) is inserted through the vocal cords and into the trachea, cuff inflated to minimal air leak (10 mL initially until patient stabilizes), and placement confirmed through capnometry or esophageal detection devices. The correct depth of insertion is verified: 21 cm (female), 23 cm (male). After insertion, the tube is secured.

> **Review Video: Mechanical Ventilation**
> Visit mometrix.com/academy and enter code: 679637

RAPID SEQUENCE INTUBATION (RSI)

Rapid sequence intubation (RSI) is the simultaneous giving of a sedative and a paralytic in order to facilitate emergency intubation and is considered to be the standard of care for emergency airway management (except in patients with anticipated difficult intubation or in those with contraindications to sedatives/paralytics).

Initial preparation includes inserting 2 IV lines and establishing cardiac monitoring, oximetry, and capnography. The patient should be preoxygenated (100%) for at least 3 minutes, but without pressure ventilation that may cause aspiration of stomach contents. Procedure includes:

- **Induction agent**: Thiopental, ketamine, etomidate, propofol
- **Paralysis**: Succinylcholine, rocuronium, other NMBAs
- **Sellick's maneuver** (pressure applied externally with thumb and index finger to cricoid) to close off the esophagus and prevent aspiration
- **Suction** to clear mouth if necessary
- **Laryngoscopy** to visual vocal cords
- **EET** inserted, cuff inflated, and ETT secured

Proper placement verified by capnometer or capnograph. Breath sounds should be auscultated. Post intubation chest x-ray to assess depth of tube and check for any trauma or issue. Induction agents and use of additional sedation may vary from one institution to another, but the primary goal is to safely anesthetize and intubate while preventing regurgitation of stomach contents.

CONFIRMING CORRECT PLACEMENT OF ENDOTRACHEAL TUBES

There are a number of methods to **confirm correct placement** of endotracheal tubes. Clinical assessment alone is not adequate.

- **Capnometry** utilizes an end-tidal CO_2 ($ETCO_2$) detector that measures the concentration of CO_2 in expired air, usually through pH sensitive paper that changes color (commonly purple to yellow). The capnometer is attached to the ETT and a bag-valve-mask (BVM) ventilator is also attached. The patient is provided 6 ventilations and the CO_2 concentration is checked.
- **Capnography** is attached to the ETT and provides a waveform graph, showing the varying concentrations of CO_2 in real time throughout each ventilation (with increased CO_2 on expiration) and can indicate changes in respiratory status.
- **Esophageal detection devices** fit over the end of the ETT so that a large syringe can be used to attempt to aspirate. If the ETT is in the esophagus, the walls collapse on aspiration and resistance occurs, whereas the syringe fills with air if the ETT is in the trachea. A self-inflating bulb (Ellik® device) may also be used.
- **Chest x-ray** provides visual confirmation of placement.

VENTILATOR MANAGEMENT

There are many types of ventilators now in use, and the specific directions for each type must be followed carefully, but there are general principles that apply to all **ventilator management**. The following should be monitored:

- **Type of ventilation:** Volume-cycled, pressure-cycled, negative-pressure, HFJV, HFOV, CPAP, Bi-PAP
- **Control mode**: Controlled ventilation, assisted ventilation, synchronized intermittent mandatory (allows spontaneous breaths between ventilator-controlled inhalation/exhalation), positive end-expiratory pressure (PEEP), CPAP, Bi-PAP
- **Tidal volume** (TV) range should be set in relation to respiratory rate
- **Inspiratory-expiratory ratio** (I:E) usually ranges from 1:2-1:5, but may vary
- **Respiratory rate** will depend upon TV and $PaCO_2$ target
- **Fraction of inspired oxygen** (FiO_2) [percentage of oxygen in the inspired air], usually ranging from 21-100%, usually maintained <40% to avoid toxicity
- **Sensitivity** determines the effort needed to trigger inspiration
- **Pressure** controls the pressure exerted in delivering TV
- **Rate of flow** controls the L/min speed of TV

HIGH FREQUENCY JET VENTILATION

High frequency jet ventilation (HFJV) (Life Pulse®) directs a high velocity stream of air into the lungs in a long spiraling spike that forces carbon dioxide against the walls, penetrating dead space and providing gas exchange by using small tidal volumes of 1-3 mL/kg, much smaller than with conventional mechanical ventilation. Because the jet stream technology is effective for short distances, the valve and pressure transducer must be placed by the person's head. Inhalation is controlled while expiration is passive, but the rate of respiration is up to 11 per second ("panting" respirations). HFJV may be used in conjunction with low-pressure conventional ventilation to increase flow to alveoli. HFJV reduces barotrauma because of the low tidal volume and low pressure. HFJV is used for numerous conditions, including evolving chronic lung disease, pulmonary interstitial emphysema, bronchopulmonary dysplasia, and hypoxemic respiratory failure. It reduces mean airway pressure (MAP) and the oxygenation index. Treatment with HFJV may reduce the need for ECMO.

HIGH FREQUENCY OSCILLATORY VENTILATION

High frequency oscillatory ventilation (HFOV) provides pressurized ventilation with tidal volumes approximately equal to dead space at about 150 breaths per minutes (BPM). Pressure is usually higher with HFOV than HFJV in order to maintain expansion of the alveoli and to keep the airway open during gas exchange. Oxygenation is regulated separately. HFOV has both an active inspiration and expiration, so the respiratory cycle is completely controlled. HFOV reduces pulmonary vascular resistance and improves ventilation-perfusion matching and oxygenation without injuring the lung, reducing the risk of barotrauma. HFOV is used for respiratory distress syndrome, persistent pulmonary hypertension, more commonly for infants and children, but there is increasing interest in using HFOV with adults because of the smaller tidal volume that prevents overinflation of the lungs and atelectasis of those with ARDS.

POSITIVE PRESSURE VENTILATORS

Positive pressure ventilators assist respiration by applying pressure directly to the airway, inflating the lungs, forcing expansion of the alveoli, and facilitating gas exchange. Generally, endotracheal intubation or tracheostomy is necessary to maintain positive pressure ventilation for extended periods. There are 3 basic kinds of positive pressure ventilators:

- **Pressure cycled:** This type of ventilation is usually used for short-term treatment in adolescents or adults. The IPPB machine is the most common type. This delivers a flow of air to a preset pressure and then cycles off. Airway resistance or changes in compliance can affect volume of air and may compromise ventilation.
- **Time cycled**: This type of ventilation regulates the volume of air the patient receives by controlling the length of inspiration and the flow rate.
- **Volume cycled**: This type of ventilation provides a preset flow of pressurized air during inspiration and then cycles off and allows passive expiration, providing a fairly consistent volume of air.

TRACHEOSTOMY

Tracheostomy, surgical tracheal opening, may be utilized for mechanical ventilation. Tracheostomy tubes are inserted directly into an opening in the trachea to provide a conduit and maintain the opening. Tracheostomy tubes are usually silastic or plastic, and may have permanent of disposable inner cannulas. The tube is secured with ties around the neck. Because the air entering the lungs through the tracheostomy bypasses the warming and moistening effects of the upper airway, air is humidified through a room humidifier or through delivery of humidified air through a special mask or mechanical ventilation. The patient with a tracheostomy must have continuous monitoring of vital signs and respiratory status to ensure patency of tracheostomy. The inner cannula should be cleaned/replaced regularly (every 8-24 hours and PRN). Regular suctioning is needed, especially initially, to remove secretions:

- Suction catheter should be 50% the size of the tracheostomy tube to allow ventilation during suctioning
- Vacuum pressure: 80-100 mmHg
- Catheter should only be inserted ≤0.5 cm beyond tube to avoid damage to tissues or perforation
- Catheter should be inserted without suction and intermittent suction on withdrawal

VENTILATION-INDUCED LUNG INJURY

Ventilation-induced lung injury (VILI) is damage caused by mechanical ventilation. It is common in acute distress syndrome (ARDS) but can affect any mechanically ventilated patient. VILI comprises four interrelated elements:

- **Barotrauma**: Damage to the lung caused by excessive pressure
- **Volutrauma**: Alveolar damage related to high tidal volume ventilation
- **Atelectotrauma**: Injury caused by repetitive forced opening and closing of alveoli
- **Biotrauma**: Inflammatory response

In VILI, essentially the increased pressure and tidal volume over-distends the alveoli, which rupture, and air moves into the interstitial tissue resulting in pulmonary interstitial emphysema. With continued ventilation, the air in the interstitium moves into the subcutaneous tissue and may result in pneumopericardium and pneumomediastinum, or rupture the pleural sac which can cause tension pneumothorax and mediastinal shift, which can cause respiratory failure and cardiac arrest. VILI has caused a change in ventilation procedures with lower tidal volumes and pressures used as well as newer forms of ventilation, HFJV and HFOV, preferred to traditional mechanical ventilation for many patients.

PREVENTING COMPLICATIONS FROM VENTILATORS

Methods to prevent complications from mechanical ventilation ("ventilator bundle") include:

- Elevate patient's head and chest to 30° to prevent aspiration and ventilation-associated pneumonia.
- Reposition patient every 2 hours.
- Provide DVT prophylaxis, such as external compression support and/or heparin (5000 u sq 2-3 times daily).
- Administer famotidine or pantoprazole PO/IV daily to prevent gastrointestinal stress-ulcers/bleeding.
- Decrease and eliminate sedation/analgesia as soon as possible—regular sedation vacations to assess neurological status.
- Follow careful protocols for pressure settings to prevent barotrauma. Tidal volumes are usually maintained at 8-12 mL/kg PBW (per AACN guidelines), but in incidences of high probability of ARDS, volumes should be less (6 mL/kg) to avoid lung injury.
- Monitor for pneumothorax or evidence of barotrauma.
- Conduct nutritional assessment (including lab tests) to prevent malnutrition.
- Monitor intake and output carefully and administer IV fluids to prevent dehydration.
- Do daily spontaneous breathing trials and discontinue ventilation as soon as possible.

VENTILATOR WEANING

Ventilator weaning has three phases: Changing settings of the ventilator to allow the patient to demonstrate the ability to breath on their own (standby mode), extubation, and finally removal of supportive oxygen. Criteria for ventilator weaning include:

- Vital capacity 10-15 mL/kg
- Maximum (negative) inspiratory pressure of at least -20 cmH$_2$O
- Tidal volume (TV) of 7-9 mL/kg
- Minute ventilation of about 6L/min (Respiratory rate x TV)
- Rapid shallow breathing index <100 breaths/min/L
- PaO$_2$ >60 mmHg
- FiO$_2$ <40%

If these criteria are met and the patient passes a spontaneous breathing trial (SBT), then extubation can be done. Various protocols are followed in weaning patients off of ventilators, including the use of intermittent mandatory ventilation (IMV) and synchronized intermittent mandatory ventilation (SIMV), which can be used with pressure support ventilation (PSV).

Criteria for oxygen weaning:

- FiO$_2$ reduced until PaO$_2$ 70-100 mmHg on room air
- Supplemental O$_2$ necessary with PaO$_2$<70 mmHg (Medicare requires PaO$_2$ 55 mmHg for reimbursement for home oxygen use)

SPONTANEOUS BREATHING TRIAL AS PREPARATION FOR EXTUBATION

A spontaneous breathing trial (SBT) is when a patient is taken off mechanical ventilation while remaining intubated (usually by changing the ventilator settings to CPAP) for a short period of time to assess readiness to extubate. SBT should be used prior to extubating a patient if the patient is not agitated and has no evidence of myocardial ischemia or increased ICP. The patient should exhibit some spontaneous triggering of respirations and should not be receiving large doses of vasopressor or inotropic agent. SpO_2 should be ≥88% with FiO_2 of 0.50 and PEEP at 7.5 cmH_2O prior to the SBT. The SBT should be done in the morning for a prescribed period (usually 30-120 minutes). The ventilator rate is adjusted to 0 and pressure support decreased to 0–7. The SBT should be discontinued if the following occur:

- Respiratory rate >35 or <8 for at least 5 minutes
- Mental status changes
- SpO_2 <88% for >15 minutes
- Respiratory distress (HR >130 BPM or <60 BPM, marked dyspnea, diaphoresis, increased use of accessory respiratory muscles, respiratory arrest)

Patients who pass the SBT have an 85-90% chance of breathing successfully after extubation. Patients who repeatedly fail daily SBT may require tracheostomy.

FAILURE TO WEAN FROM MECHANICAL VENTILATION

Failure to wean from mechanical ventilation can occur in approximately 20-30% of ventilated patients. Many factors affect a patient's ability to wean from mechanical ventilation including physical, psychological, and situational factors. Before discontinuation of ventilation can be considered, the patient must be able to protect his/her airway, be hemodynamically stable and have resolution of the clinical problem that initiated the need for mechanical ventilation. Weaning protocols use clinical criteria such as oxygen saturation, blood pressure, respiratory rate, and tidal volume to determine the patient's tolerance of lessening mechanical ventilator support. Failure to wean is demonstrated by multiple daily spontaneous breathing trial failures or the need for reintubation within 48 hours of extubation. Failure to resolve the clinical problem(s) that initiated mechanical ventilation, insufficient ventilator drive, respiratory muscle weakness, co-morbidities, and/or the development of new clinical problems (e.g., infection) may contribute to the inability to wean.

Signs and symptoms: Decreased tidal volume, increased respiratory rate, increased $PaCO_2$, oxygen desaturation, anxiety, diaphoresis, fatigue, changes in blood pressure or heart rate, mental status changes, and hemodynamic changes.

Treatment: The initial treatment strategy for patients who experience a dysfunctional ventilator weaning response is identification and treatment of the underlying cause(s) of the weaning failure. In addition, other treatment strategies may include psychological preparation of the patient for further weaning attempts, readiness testing and respiratory muscle training.

SEDATION/ANALGESIA WITH MECHANICAL VENTILATION

Patients intubated for mechanical ventilation are usually given **sedation and/or analgesia** initially, but medications should be reduced and given in boluses rather than with continuous IV drip with a goal of stopping sedation as it prolongs ventilation time. Typical sedatives include midazolam, propofol, and lorazepam. Narcotic analgesics include fentanyl and morphine sulfate. Uses of sedation include:

- Controlling agitation and excessive movement that may interfere with ventilation
- Reduce pain and discomfort associated with ventilation
- Control respiratory distress

Triglyceride levels must be checked periodically if propofol is administered for more than 24–48 hours. Neuromuscular blocking agents are rarely used because they may cause long-term weakness and increase length of ventilation although they may be indicated in some cases, such as with

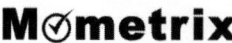

excessive shivering or cardiac arrest. Many patients are able to tolerate mechanical ventilation without sedation, and sedation should always be decreased to the minimal amount necessary as excess sedation may delay extubation. An ideal level of sedation will keep the patient calm and compliant with the ventilator but still alert and able to follow commands.

CONSCIOUS SEDATION

Conscious sedation is used to decrease sensations of pain and awareness caused by a surgical or invasive procedure, such a biopsy, chest tube insertion, fracture repair, and endoscopy. It is also used during presurgical preparations, such as insertion of central lines, catheters, and use of cooling blankets. Conscious sedation uses a combination of analgesia and sedation so that patients can remain responsive and follow verbal cues but have a brief amnesia preventing recall of the procedures. The patient must be monitored carefully, including pulse oximetry, during this type of sedation. The most commonly used drugs include:

- Midazolam (Versed®): This is a short-acting water-soluble sedative, with onset of 1-5 minutes, peaking in 30, and duration usually about 1 hour (up to 6 hours).
- Fentanyl: This is a short-acting opioid with immediate onset, peaking in 10-15 minutes and with a duration of about 20-45 minutes. Monitor respiratory function.

The fentanyl/midazolam combination provides both sedation and pain control. Conscious sedation usually requires 6 hours fasting prior to administration.

THERAPEUTIC GASES

Carbon dioxide is a potent stimulator of respirations, but it is rarely used therapeutically because it can depress respirations if hypercarbia or respiratory acidosis is present. CO_2 may be administered at times as part of anesthesia, but it is most commonly used for insufflation for laparoscopic/endoscopic procedures.

Nitric oxide (NO) is used as a pulmonary vessel dilator to improve oxygenation by decreasing pulmonary artery pressure and pulmonary vascular resistance. NO is FDA-approved for use for neonatal PPH but is sometimes used for adults, although studies have not shown it an effective treatment for ARDS. NO should be delivered at 0.1-50 ppm to avoid toxicity that can occur over 50 ppm. Toxic reactions include methemoglobinemia and platelet inhibition with resultant bleeding.

Heliox is helium mixed with oxygen that is used to reduce airway resistance during mechanical ventilation and for pulmonary function tests. Heliox may also be used to treat respiratory obstruction and is used during laser surgery on the airway because it readily conducts heat away from the surgical site, reducing tissue damage. Heliox is sometimes used for COPD patients as it increases hyperventilation and reduces carbon dioxide levels.

Renal

PROCEDURES FOR INSERTION AND REMOVAL OF URINARY CATHETER

Procedure for inserting and removing a urinary catheter:

1. Gather supplies (included in a urinary catheter insertion kit), perform hand hygiene, place a waterproof pad under the patient, and ensure that the light source is adequate to view the urinary meatus.
2. Place females in supine position with knees flexed and males in supine position.
3. Apply gloves and wash the perineal area with facility provided cleanser (sometimes included in the outside of the urinary catheter kit) and allow to dry.
4. Remove gloves and wash hands.
5. Using aseptic technique, place the catheter kit between the patient's legs, open the kit touching only the corners of the drape that wraps around the kit.
6. Apply sterile gloves.
7. Apply sterile drapes to the patient.
8. Following the steps provided with the kit, place the lubricant into the appropriate section of tray, remove the catheter from its plastic and place the tip into the lubricant, and pour iodine over the three cleansing swabs (if they do not come impregnated with iodine already). Attach the 10-cc syringe (filled with sterile water) to the appropriate port of the catheter.
9. Cleanse the urethral meatus with the iodine impregnated swabs.
10. Using the nondominant hand, hold the penis or open the labia to observe the urethral meatus. This hand now becomes "dirty" and cannot be used to touch the catheter.
11. Using the dominant hand, insert catheter with the drainage end attached to the collection bag. Insert until urine flows freely, advancing a little further after that point.
12. Inflate the balloon using the 10-cc sterile water syringe, and ensure the catheter is secure.
13. Secure the catheter to the patient's leg and hang the collection bag below the level of the patient. Secure any tubing to the bed and ensure no kinking is present.

Removal: Straight catheter—remove by pulling out slowly. To remove indwelling catheter, deflate the balloon using the appropriate port and gently pull the catheter out.

REDUCING INFECTION RISKS ASSOCIATED WITH URINARY CATHETERS

Strategies for reducing infection risks associated with urinary catheters include:

- Using **aseptic technique** for both the straight and indwelling catheter insertion
- **Limiting catheter use** by establishing protocols for use, duration, and removal; training staff; issuing reminders to physicians; using straight catheterizations rather than indwelling; using ultrasound to scan the bladder; and using condom catheters
- Utilizing **closed-drainage systems** for indwelling catheters
- **Avoiding irrigation** unless required for diagnosis or treatment
- Using **sampling port** for specimens rather than disconnecting catheter and tubing
- Maintaining **proper urinary flow** by proper positioning, securing of tubing and drainage bag, and keeping the drainage bag below the level of the bladder
- **Changing catheters** only when medically needed
- **Cleansing external meatal area** gently each day, manipulating the catheter as little as possible
- Avoiding placing catheterized patients adjacent to those infected or colonized with antibiotic-resistant bacteria to reduce **cross-contamination**

RENAL REPLACEMENT THERAPY

PERITONEAL DIALYSIS

Renal dialysis is used primarily for those who have progressed from renal insufficiency to uremia with end-stage renal disease (ESRD). It may also be temporarily for acute conditions. People can be maintained on dialysis, but there are many complications associated with dialysis, so many people are considered for renal transplantation. There are a number of different approaches to **peritoneal dialysis:**

- **Peritoneal dialysis:** An indwelling catheter is inserted surgically into the peritoneal cavity with a subcutaneous tunnel and a Dacron cuff to prevent infection. Sterile dialysate solution is slowly instilled through gravity, remains for a prescribed length of time, and is then drained and discarded.
- **Continuous ambulatory peritoneal dialysis:** a series of exchange cycles is repeated 24 hours a day.
- **Continuous cyclic peritoneal dialysis:** a prolonged period of retaining fluid occurs during the day with drainage at night.

Peritoneal dialysis may be used for those who want to be more independent, don't live near a dialysis center, or want fewer dietary restrictions.

> **Review Video: End-Stage Renal Disease**
> Visit mometrix.com/academy and enter code: 869617

HEMODIALYSIS

Hemodialysis, the most common type of dialysis, is used for both short-term dialysis and long-term for those with ESRD. Treatments are usually done three times weekly for 3-4 hours or daily dialysis with treatment either during the night or in short daily periods. **Hemodialysis** is often done for those who can't manage peritoneal dialysis or who live near a dialysis center, but it does interfere with work or school attendance and requires strict dietary and fluid restrictions between treatments. Short daily dialysis allows more independence, and increased costs may be offset by lower morbidity. A vascular access device, such as a catheter, fistula, or graft, must be established for hemodialysis, and heparin is used to prevent clotting. With hemodialysis, blood is circulated outside of the body through a dialyzer (a synthetic semipermeable membrane), which filters the blood. There are many different types of dialyzers. High flux dialyzers use a highly permeable membrane that shortens the duration of treatment and decreases the need for heparin.

CONTINUOUS RENAL REPLACEMENT THERAPY

Continuous renal replacement therapy (CRRT) circulates the blood by hydrostatic pressure through a semipermeable membrane. It is used in critical care and can be instituted quickly:

- **Continuous arteriovenous hemofiltration** (CAVH) circulates blood from an artery (usually the femoral) to a hemofilter using only arterial pressure and not a blood pump. The filtered blood is then returned to the patient's venous system, often with added fluids to offset those lost. Only the fluid is filtered.
- **Continuous arteriovenous hemodialysis** (CAVHD) is similar to CAVH except that dialysate circulates on one side of the semipermeable membrane to increase the clearance of urea.

- **Continuous venovenous hemofiltration** (CVVH) pumps blood through a double-lumen venous catheter to a hemofilter, which returns the blood to the patient in the same catheter. It provides continuous slow removal of fluid, is better tolerated with unstable patients, and doesn't require arterial access.
- **Continuous venovenous hemodialysis** is similar to CVVH but uses a dialysate to increase the clearance of uremic toxins.

DIALYSIS COMPLICATIONS

There are many complications associated with dialysis, especially when used for long-term treatment:

- **Hemodialysis**: Long-term use promotes atherosclerosis and cardiovascular disease. Anemia and fatigue are common, as are infections related to access devices or contamination of equipment. Some experience hypotension and muscle cramping during treatment. Dysrhythmias may occur. Some may exhibit dialysis disequilibrium from cerebral fluid shifts, causing headaches, nausea and vomiting, and alterations of consciousness.
- **Peritoneal dialysis:** Most complications are minor, but it can lead to peritonitis, which requires removal of the catheter if antibiotic therapy is not successful in clearing the infection within 4 days. There may be leakage of the dialysate around the catheter. Bleeding may occur, especially in females who are menstruating as blood is pulled from the uterus through the fallopian tubes. Abdominal hernias may occur with long use. Some may have anorexia from the feeling of fullness or a sweet taste in the mouth from the absorption of glucose.

Multisystem Procedures and Interventions

TARGETED TEMPERATURE MANAGEMENT

Targeted temperature management (previously referred to as therapeutic hypothermia) is used to reduce ischemic tissue damage associated with cardiac arrest, ischemic stroke, traumatic brain/spinal cord injury, neurogenic fever, and subsequent coma (3 on Glasgow scale). Reducing the body's temperature to below normal range has a neuroprotective effect by making cell membranes less permeable, thus reducing neurologic edema and damage. Hypothermia should be initiated immediately after an ischemic event if possible, but some benefit remains up to 6 hours. Hypothermia to 33 °C may be induced by cooled saline through a femoral catheter, reducing temperature 1.5-2.0 °C/hr by an electronic control unit. Hypothermic water blankets covering ≥80% of the body's surface can also lower body temperature. In some cases, both a femoral cooling catheter and a water blanket are used for rapid reduction of temperature. Rectal probes are used to measure core temperature, but Foley temperature catheters are more common. Desflurane or meperidine is given to reduce the shivering response. Hypothermia increases risk of bleeding (decreased clotting time), infection (due to impairing leukocyte function and introducing catheters), arrhythmias, hyperglycemia, and DVT. Rewarming is done slowly at 0.5-1.0 °C/hr. through warmed intravenous fluids, warm humidified air, and/or warming blanket. The warming process is a critical time, as it causes potassium to be moved from extracellular to intracellular spaces and the patient's electrolyte levels must be monitored regularly.

CONTINUOUS TEMPERATURE MONITORING

Continuous temperature monitoring may be carried out through various means:

- Pulmonary artery catheter (most accurate but generally not recommended because of invasiveness and potential for complications)
- Rectal or Foley temperature probes
- Skin probes
- Wearable Bluetooth monitors (patch applied to the skin), which transmit information to an external monitor or the patient's electronic health record. (For external temperature monitoring, the device must be applied properly and for the correct duration of time [e.g., the TempTraQ® wearable patch is applied in the underarm area and measures temperature for 72 hours].)

Indications for continuous temperature monitoring include:

- Skin flap transplantation—to assess perfusion
- Brain injury—to assess thermoregulation
- Therapeutic hypothermia—for cardiac arrest or post-cardiac surgery
- Malignant hyperthermia
- Immunocompromised patients—to assess for signs of infection
- Critically ill patients—at risk for temperature dysregulation

PALLIATIVE AND END-OF-LIFE CARE

GRIEF

Grief is an emotional response to a **loss** that begins at the time a loss is anticipated and continues on an individual timetable. While there are identifiable stages or tasks, it is not an orderly and predictable process. It involves overcoming anger, disbelief, guilt, and a myriad of related emotions. The grieving individual may move back and forth between stages or experience several emotions at any given time. Each person's grief response is unique to their own coping patterns, stress levels, age, gender, belief system, and previous experiences with loss.

KUBLER-ROSS'S FIVE STAGES OF GRIEF

Kubler-Ross taught the medical and nursing community that the dying patient and family welcomes open, honest discussion of the dying process and felt that there were certain **stages** that patients and family go through. The stages may not occur in order, but may vary or some may be skipped. Stages include:

- **Denial**: The person denies the diagnosis and tries to pretend it isn't true. During this time, the person may seek a second opinion or alternative therapies. They may use denial until they are better able to emotionally cope with the reality of the disease or changes that need to be made. Patients may also wish to save family and friends from pain and worry. Both patients and family may use denial as a coping mechanism when they feel overwhelmed by the reality of the disease and threatened losses.
- **Anger**: The person is angry about the situation and may focus that rage on anyone.
- **Bargaining**: The person attempts to make deals with a higher power to secure a better outcome to their situation.
- **Depression**: The person anticipates the loss and the changes it will bring with a sense of sadness and grief.
- **Acceptance**: The person accepts the impending death and is ready to face it as it approaches. The patient may begin to withdraw from interests and family.

> **Review Video: The Five Stages of Grief**
> Visit mometrix.com/academy and enter code: 648794

PALLIATIVE AND HOSPICE CARE

Palliative care attempts to make the rest of the patient's life as comfortable as possible by treating distressing symptoms to keep them controlled. It does not attempt to cure but only to control discomfort caused by the disease. Palliative care does not require terminal illness/prognosis and can be implemented for any patient with chronic disease and suffering.

Hospice care uses palliative care as it supports the patient and family through the dying process. Hospice teams support the daily needs of the patient and family and provide needed equipment, medical expertise, and medications to control symptoms. They offer spiritual, psychological, and social support to the patient and family as needed and desired. Assistance with end-of-life planning is given to help the patient and family accomplish goals important to them. Bereavement support is also given. The team consists of the attending physician, hospice physician advisor, nurses, social worker, clergy, hospice aides, and volunteers. Hospice care is given in the home when the patient has family who are willing to assume care with the assistance of the hospice team. Hospice care also occurs in hospice facilities, hospitals, and extended care facilities. To qualify for Hospice care, the patient must be deemed terminal and given a 6-month or less life expectancy by two separate physicians. Should the patient survive 6 months in hospice, they can be extended for two 90-day periods, and then an unlimited number of 60-day periods per physician order.

WHO PAIN LADDER

The WHO pain ladder was developed as an algorithm for treating pain through medications with progressively increasing potency. The approach can be used effectively with both adult and pediatric patients. Beginning with the least potent medication option, each step adds a stronger analgesic until optimum pain relief is reached.

The **WHO pain ladder** has three steps.

- **Step 1**: The patient is given a non-opioid medication which may be used alone or in conjunction with other adjuvant therapies.
- **Step 2**: If the patient reports no change in the pain level, mild- to moderate-level pain-relieving opioids are introduced along with adjuvants if they have not been previously introduced.
- **Step 3**: Uncontrolled pain is then treated with opioids for moderate to severe pain. Adjuvants may also be continued.

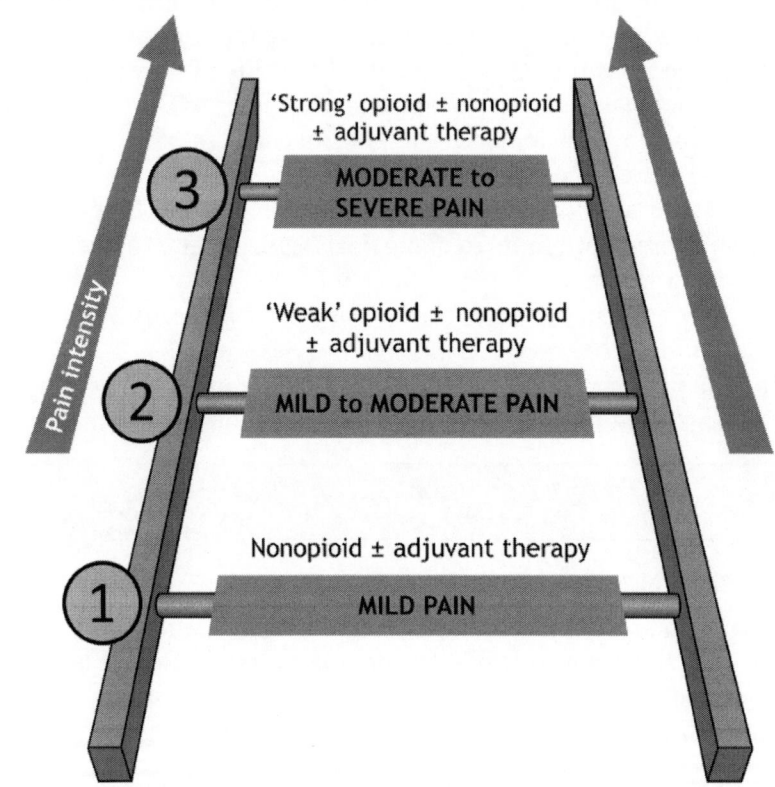

Review Video: Adjuvants
Visit mometrix.com/academy and enter code: 178200

Monitoring and Diagnostics

Cardiovascular

ASSESSMENT OF THE CARDIOVASCULAR SYSTEM

Cardiovascular assessment includes questioning the patient for any family history of death at a young age or other cardiovascular diseases. Elderly African-American males are at highest risk for cardiovascular problems. One must question the patient about edema, chest pain, dyspnea, fatigue, vertigo, syncope or other changes in consciousness, weight gain, and leg cramps or pain. If chest pain is a symptom, one must ask about the intensity, timing, location, any radiation, quality, meaning to the patient, factors that aggravate or alleviate the pain, nausea, dyspnea, diaphoresis, or any other accompanying symptoms. Physical assessment includes assessment of vital signs, heart and lung sounds, skin assessment, radial, popliteal, and pedal pulses, circulation and sensation of extremities, and auscultation of the aorta, renal, iliac, and femoral arteries for bruits. Blood should be taken for a lipid profile and electrolytes. The patient must be helped to modify risk factors such as hypertension, smoking, diabetes, obesity, hyperlipidemia, inactivity, and stress.

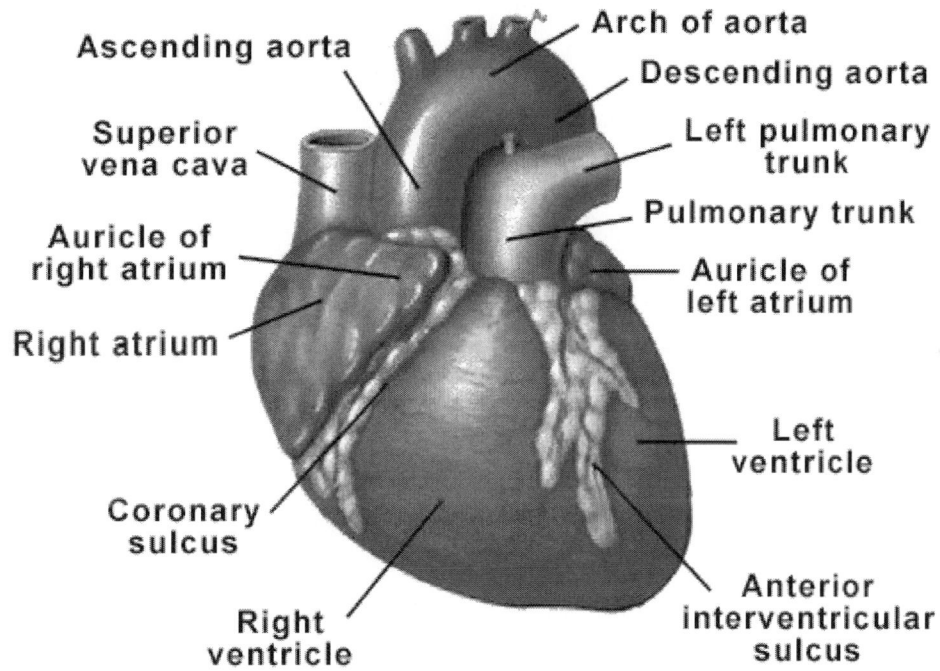

Review Video: **Cardiovascular Assessment**
Visit mometrix.com/academy and enter code: 323076

Review Video: **Functions of the Circulatory System**
Visit mometrix.com/academy and enter code: 376581

Review Video: **Heart Blood Flow**
Visit mometrix.com/academy and enter code: 783139

HEMODYNAMIC MONITORING

MAP

The MAP **(mean arterial pressure)** is most commonly used to evaluate perfusion as it shows pressure throughout the cardiac cycle. Systole is one-third and diastole two-thirds of the normal cardiac cycle. The MAP for a blood pressure of 120/60 is calculated as follows:

$$MAP = \frac{\text{Diastole} \times 2 + \text{Systole}}{3}$$

$$MAP = \frac{60 \times 2 + 120}{3} = \frac{240}{3} = 80$$

Normal range for mean arterial pressure is 70-100 mmHg. A MAP of greater than 60 mmHg is required to perfuse vital organs, including the heart, brain, and kidneys.

ARTERIAL LINE INSERTION

Indications for an **arterial line** include hemodynamic instability, frequent ABG monitoring, placement of IABP, monitoring arterial pressure, and medication administration when venous access cannot be obtained. Sterile technique is utilized for arterial line insertion. Insertions sites include radial (most common), femoral (second choice), brachial, or dorsalis pedis arteries.
Procedure:

- Verify adequate perfusion and position.
    - Radial: Perform modified Allen test and position wrist in dorsiflexion with an arm board.
    - Femoral: Place the patient in a supine position with the leg on the insertion side slightly abducted and extended.
- Prep and drape. Apply 1% lidocaine if the patient is conscious.
- Insert needle.
    - Over-the-needle catheter insertion: Needle is inserted at a 30-45° degree angle and decreased to a 10-15° angle when blood returns, catheter advanced into vessel, needle removed, and catheter connected to transducer.
    - Over-wire catheter insertion: Needle is inserted into the artery at a 30-45° angle until blood returns. A wire is then inserted and advanced through the needle, and needle removed, leaving the wire in place. A catheter is then advanced over the wire, wire removed, and catheter connected to transducer system.
- A small incision is made at insertion site and catheter sutured into place.

Complications include bleeding, coagulopathy, thrombosis (especially with larger catheters or smaller arteries), advanced atherosclerosis, and infection.

> **Review Video: Nursing Care of Arterial Lines**
> Visit mometrix.com/academy and enter code: 561047

OXYGEN SATURATION AS IT RELATES TO HEMODYNAMIC STATUS

Hemodynamic monitoring includes monitoring **oxygen saturation** levels, which must be maintained for proper cardiac function. The central venous catheter often has an oxygen sensor at the tip to monitor oxygen saturation in the right atrium. If the catheter tip is located near the renal veins, this can cause an increase in right atrial oxygen saturation; and near the coronary sinus, a decrease.

- Increased oxygen saturation may result from left atrial to right atrial shunt, abnormal pulmonary venous return, increased delivery of oxygen or decrease in extraction of oxygen.
- Decreased oxygen saturation may be related to low cardiac output with an increase in oxygen extraction or decrease in arterial oxygen saturation with normal differences in the atrial and ventricular oxygen saturation.

CARDIAC OUTPUT

Cardiac output (CO) is the amount of blood pumped through the ventricles during a specified period. Normal cardiac output is about 5 liters per minutes at rest for an adult. Under exercise or stress, this volume may multiply 3 or 4 times with concomitant changes in the heart rate (HR) and stroke volume (SV). The basic formulation for calculating cardiac output is the heart rate (HR) per minute multiplied by the stroke volume (SR), which is the amount of blood pumped through the ventricles with each contraction. The stroke volume is controlled by preload, afterload, and contractibility.

$$CO \left(\frac{mL}{min} \right) = HR \left(\frac{beats}{min} \right) \times SV \text{ (mL)}$$

The heart rate is controlled by the autonomic nervous system. Normally, if the heart rate decreases, stroke volume increases to compensate. The exception to this would be cardiomyopathies, so bradycardia results in a sharp decline in cardiac output.

CARDIAC INDEX

Cardiac index (CI) is the cardiac output (CO) divided by the body surface area (BSA). This is essentially a measure of cardiac output tailored to the individual, based on height and weight, measured in liters/min per square meter of BSA.

- Normal value: 2.2–4.0 L/min/m²

STROKE VOLUME

Stroke volume (SV) is the amount of blood pumped through the left ventricle with each contraction, minus any blood remaining inside the ventricle at the end of systole.

- Normal values: 60–70 mL
- Formula:

$$SV \text{ (mL)} = CO \left(\frac{mL}{min} \right) \div HR \left(\frac{beats}{min} \right)$$

PULMONARY VASCULAR RESISTANCE AND EJECTION FRACTION

Pulmonary vascular resistance (PVR) is the resistance in the pulmonary arteries and arterioles against which the right ventricle has to pump during contraction. It is the mean pressure in the pulmonary vascular bed divided by blood flow. If PVR increases, SV decreases.

- Normal value: 1.2–3.0 units or 100–250 dynes/sec/cm⁵

Ejection Fraction (EF) is the percentage of the total blood volume of the heart that is pumped out with each beat. Dramatically decreased values indicate heart failure.

- Normal value: 60–70%

PRELOAD AND AFTERLOAD

Preload refers to the amount of elasticity in the myocardium at the end of diastole when the ventricles are filled to their maximum volume and the stretch on the muscle fibers is the greatest. The preload value is based on the volume in the ventricles. The amount of preload (stretch) affects stroke volume because as stretch increases, the resultant contraction also increases (Frank-Starling Law). Preload may decrease because of dehydration, diuresis, or vasodilation. Preload may increase because of increased venous return, controlling fluid loss, transfusion, or intravenous fluids.

Afterload refers to the amount of systemic vascular resistance to left ventricular ejection of blood and pulmonary vascular resistance to right ventricular ejection of blood. Determinants of afterload include the size and elasticity of the great vessels and the functioning of the pulmonic and aortic valves. Afterload increases with hypertension, stenotic valves, and vasoconstriction.

MINIMALLY/NON-INVASIVE HEMODYNAMIC MONITORING

Hemodynamic monitoring and evaluation of cardiac function is an important component of the care of the critically ill patient. **Minimally or non-invasive** alternatives to traditional invasive means of hemodynamic monitoring (such as the use of a pulmonary artery catheter) include esophageal Doppler, arterial pressure based cardiac output monitoring, and impedance cardiography. **Esophageal Doppler** is a minimally invasive option used in surgical patients to monitor descending aortic blood flow and estimate cardiac output. A probe is inserted into the esophagus and then connected to a monitor, where waveform shapes produced by aortic blood flow are displayed.

Arterial pressure based cardiac output monitors (APCO's) use an algorithm to estimate cardiac output through the analysis of the arterial pressure waveform. The radial or femoral artery is accessed using a standard arterial catheter and no external calibration is needed.

Impedance cardiography is a non-invasive method of hemodynamic monitoring in which sensors placed on the body use electrical signals to measure the level of change in impedance in the thoracic fluid. A waveform is generated and is then used to calculate cardiac output and stroke volume, as well as ten additional hemodynamic parameters.

INTRAARTERIAL BLOOD PRESSURE MONITORING

Intraarterial blood pressure monitoring uses a catheter to measure systolic, diastolic, and mean arterial pressures (MAP) continuously. Before catheter insertion, collateral circulation must be assessed by Doppler or the Allen test (radial). Complications include arterial vasospasm, hematoma formation, hemorrhage (accidental disconnect), catheter occlusion, compartment syndrome, retroperitoneal bleed (femoral site), and thrombus/embolus.

Set up: The line should be connected to the monitor as well as a pressure bag set at 300 mmHg with no longer than 3 feet of stiff, noncompliant tubing to ensure accuracy. The transducer is leveled at the phlebostatic axis of the patient. The line should be kept free of any air or bubbles, and re-zeroed every four hours and with a change of patient position.

Waveform: A normal ABP waveform should be smooth and regular, with a dicrotic notch. To test, perform a "square-wave" or "Fast Flush" test; flush the line while watching the monitor. There should be a square shape, followed by two oscillations and a return to normal waves. A missing dicrotic notch indicates a blockage of some kind (thrombus, plaque, and vasospasm) or low pressure in the bag. Too many oscillations or an increased sharpness of the wave indicates under dampening and is caused by increased SVR or too long of tubing.

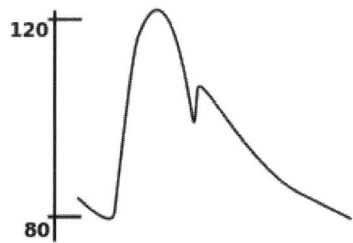

ECHOCARDIOGRAPHY

Echocardiography is a non-invasive ultrasound technology that is very useful for assessing and diagnosing anatomic heart abnormalities, blood flow, and valvular lesions:

- The **standard "2D Echo"** is used best for basic structural imaging, such as valvular lesions and assessment of pericardial disorders.
- The **transesophageal (TEE)** probe is an improved version of echocardiography, which allows better visualization of the left atrium and more precise evaluation of the valvular structure. TEE is also the best modality for evaluation of the thoracic aorta in the setting of suspected aortic dissection or aneurysm.
- **Doppler imaging** is used to measure blood flow, often in the context of velocity across a valve and a pressure gradient.
- **Bubble study** is an addition to echocardiography allowing the study to determine if there is right to left blood flow through a patent foramen ovale or a more distal intrapulmonary shunt of blood.

ELECTROCARDIOGRAM

The electrocardiogram records and shows a graphic display of the electrical activity of the heart through a number of different waveforms, complexes, and intervals:

- **P wave**: Start of electrical impulse in the sinus node and spreading through the atria, muscle depolarization
- **QRS complex**: Ventricular muscle depolarization and atrial repolarization
- **T wave**: Ventricular muscle repolarization (resting state) as cells regain negative charge
- **U wave**: Repolarization of the Purkinje fibers

A modified lead II ECG is often used to monitor basic heart rhythms and dysrhythmias:

- Typical placement of leads for 2-lead ECG is 3-5 cm inferior to the right clavicle and left lower ribcage. Typical placement for a 3-lead ECG is (RA) right arm near shoulder, (LA) V_5 position over 5th intercostal space, and (LL) left upper leg near groin.

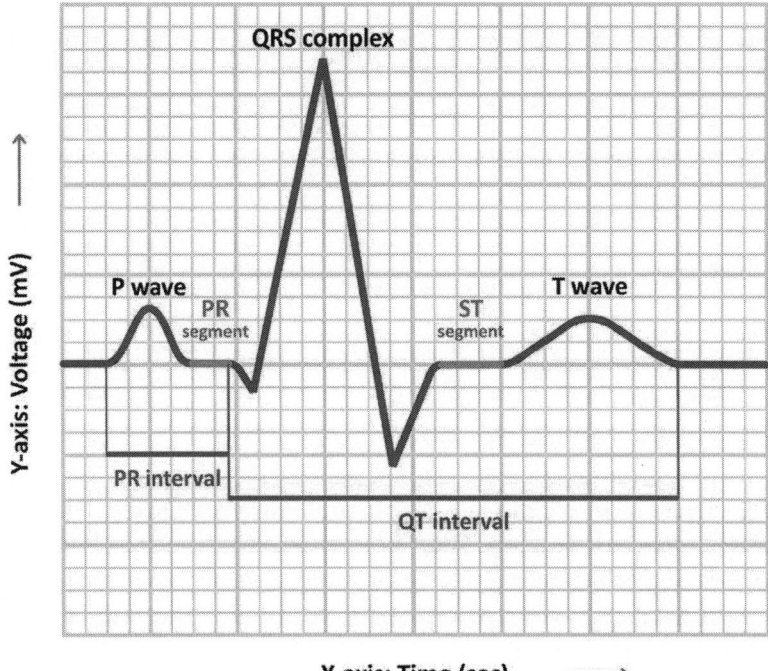

ADMINISTRATION OF 12-LEAD ECG

The electrocardiogram provides a graphic representation of the electrical activity of the heart. It is indicated for chest pain, dyspnea, syncope, acute coronary syndrome, pulmonary embolism, and possible MI. The standard **12 lead ECG** gives a picture of electrical activity from 12 perspectives through placement of 10 body leads:

- 4 limb leads are placed distally on the wrists and ankles (but may be placed more proximally if necessary).
- Precordial leads:
  - V1: Right sternal border at 4th intercostal space
  - V2: Left sternal border at 4th intercostal space
  - V3: Midway between V2 and V4
  - V4: Left midclavicular line at 5th intercostal space
  - V5: Horizontal to V4 at left anterior axillary line
  - V6: Horizontal to V5 at left midaxillary line

In some cases, additional leads may be used:

- Right-sided leads are placed on the right in a mirror image of the left leads, usually to diagnose right ventricular infarction through ST elevation.

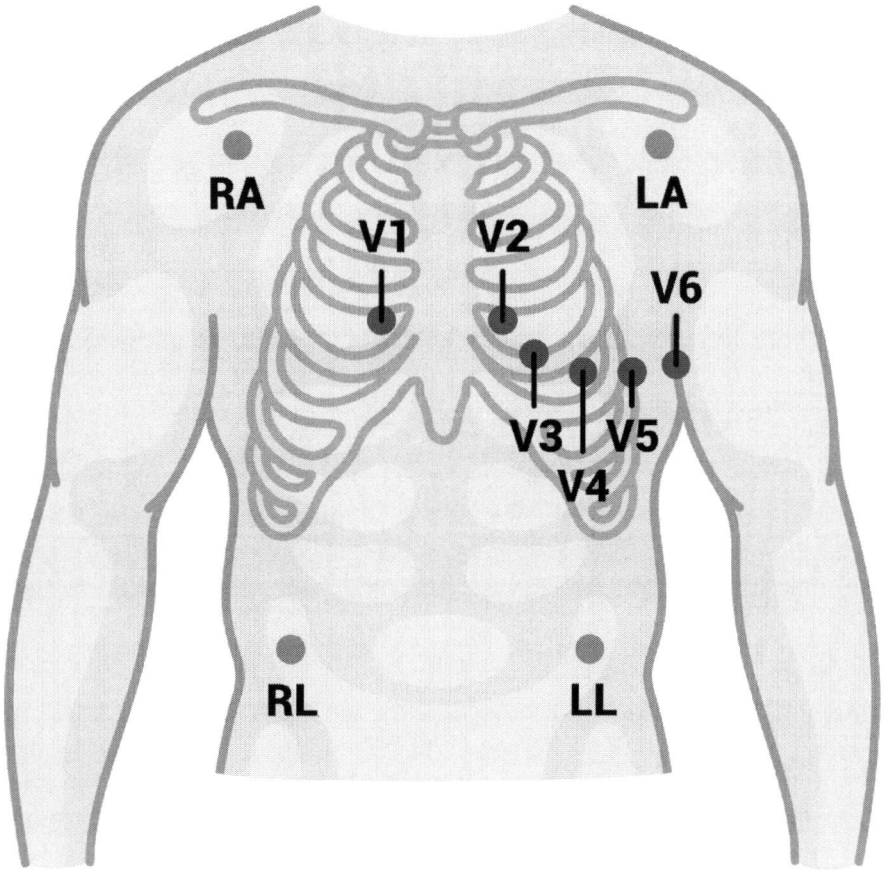

LABORATORY TESTING
CK AND CK-MB

Creatine kinase (CK) and CK-MB levels are evaluated every 6–8 hours in a suspected myocardial injury. Total CK and CK-MB (specific to cardiac cells) initially rise within the first 4–6 hours of an MI. A normal range would be 30 IU/L to 180 IU/L for CK and CK-MB totaling 0–5% of the CK level.

Assuming no further damage is sustained, peak levels (in excess of 6 times the normal range) are reached 12–24 hours after the injury. CK levels will return to normal within 3–4 days of the event. Small spikes in CK level might also occur following invasive cardiac procedures.

TROPONIN I AND T

Troponin, which is found in cardiac and skeletal muscle, is a type of protein. Both troponin I and T (isolates of troponin) are found in the myocardium, but troponin T is also found in skeletal muscle, so it is less specific than troponin I. Troponin I, therefore, may be used to detect a myocardial infarction after non-cardiac surgery and to detect acute coronary syndrome. Troponin is released into the bloodstream when injury to the tissue (such as the myocardium) occurs and causes damage to the cell membranes, as occurs with myocardial injury.

- **Troponin I** (<0.05 ng/mL): Appears in 2-6 hours, peaks at 15-20 hours and returns to normal in 5-7 days. Exhibits a second but lower peak at 60-80 hours (biphasic).
- **Troponin T** (<0.2 ng/mL): Increases 2-6 hours after MI and stays elevated. Returns to normal in 7 days. (Less specific than troponin I)

STRESS TESTING

Basic **cardiac stress testing** consists of exercise EKG testing (EET) and exercise imaging testing. The exercise imaging testing may be broken down into exercise, or "stress" echocardiography, and exercise myocardial perfusion imaging.

Exercise imaging testing is usually performed with echocardiography. Stress echocardiography is performed similarly to exercise EKG testing and also requires that the patient meet at least 85% maximum heart rate in order to attain optimum sensitivity and specificity. (The maximum heart rate formula is 220 minus the person's age.) Of note, chemicals may substitute for exercise during the "stress" portion of the test. This may be performed with dobutamine (beta-1-agonist: cannot be used after beta-blocker administration) or adenosine (causes diffuse coronary dilatation, leading to decreased perfusion pressure and unmasking of defects, and cannot be used with asthma). Stress imaging allows the study to determine the actual area of ischemia and whether or not this is a reversible defect. Additional information obtained during echocardiography is cardiac output and measurement of viability.

MYOCARDIAL PERFUSION IMAGING TECHNIQUES

Stress perfusion studies are often interchanged with stress echocardiography, as they are both good at determining areas of ischemia and reversible wall motion defects. Myocardial perfusion imaging is often performed with the administration of adenosine to induce diffuse coronary dilatation, which unmasks perfusion defects. This test is performed using either thallium 201 or technetium 99. The use of these tracers allows for more exact determination of cardiac blood flow. Basically, the ischemic areas take up fewer tracers during peak "stress" than do normal areas. If these changes persist during rest, then this area is deemed infracted. Images may be repeated in 24 hours to determine if there is an increased area of viability.

Respiratory

ASSESSMENT OF THE RESPIRATORY SYSTEM

If significant respiratory distress is present, one must stabilize the patient before doing a **respiratory history** or ask family if available:

- Question the patient about risk factors, such as smoking, exposure to smoke or other inhaled toxins, past lung problems, and allergies.
- Ask the patient about symptoms of respiratory problems, such as dyspnea, cough, sputum production, fatigue, ability to do ADLs and IADLs, and chest pain.
- Determine how long symptoms have been present, the length of periods of dyspnea, aggravating and alleviating factors, and the severity of symptoms.

When performing a **physical assessment**, one should assess vital signs, posture, pulse oximetry, check nails for clubbing, do a skin assessment, listen to lung sounds via auscultation and percussion, and look for accessory muscle use, signs of anxiety, and edema. Depending on condition, blood may be drawn for arterial blood gases, electrolytes, and CBC. Sputum cultures may be obtained.

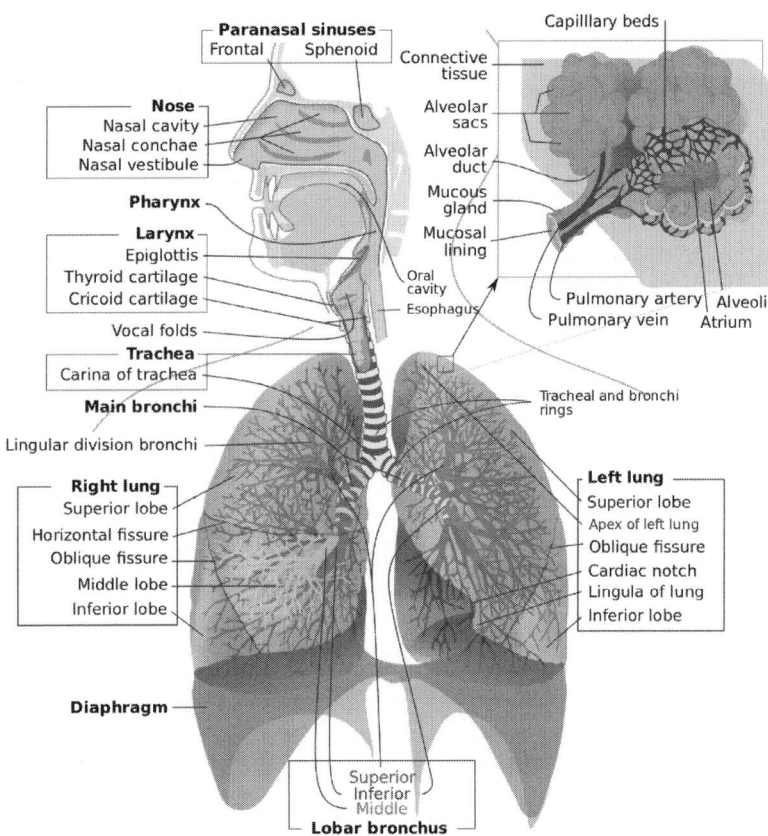

Review Video: Respiratory System
Visit mometrix.com/academy and enter code: 783075

123

ARTERIAL OXYGEN SATURATION AND VENOUS OXYGEN SATURATION

Arterial oxygen saturation (SaO_2) measures the amount of oxygen that is bound to hemoglobin and dissolved in plasma in arterial blood. It measures the degree of oxygenation produced by the lungs. A normal SaO_2 range is 90-100%. SaO_2 can be measured with a pulse oximeter probe (abbreviated SpO_2) or by drawing an arterial blood gas sample.

Venous oxygen saturations (SvO_2) measure the amount of oxygen bound to hemoglobin and dissolved within the plasma of the blood when it is returning from the body to the heart and lungs. SvO_2 measures cardiac output and tissue oxygen consumption. The normal range for SvO_2 is between 60 and 80%.

VENOUS GAS

Venous oxygen saturation (SvO_2) is measured by drawing a mixed venous gas sample from the distal port of the pulmonary artery catheter. Drawing blood from the distal port provides a sampling of blood from different parts of the body prior to be being oxygenated by the lungs. Mixed venous blood can be drawn intermittently and assessed by being sent to the lab, or it can be monitored continuously using a fiberoptic attachment on the distal tip of the catheter.

The normal range for SvO_2 is 60 to 80%, which indicates adequate cardiac output and tissue perfusion. An SvO_2 between 40 and 60% indicates inadequate tissue oxygenation. An SvO_2 less than 40% indicates a significant oxygen supply-demand imbalance; either the cardiac output is inadequate, or tissue oxygen demands are elevated.

ARTERIAL BLOOD GASES

Arterial blood gases (ABGs) are monitored to assess effectiveness of oxygenation, ventilation, and acid-base status and to determine oxygen flow rates. Partial pressure of a gas is that exerted by each gas in a mixture of gases, proportional to its concentration, based on total atmospheric pressure of 760 mmHg at sea level. Normal values include:

- Acidity/alkalinity (pH): 7.35-7.45
- Partial pressure of carbon dioxide ($PaCO_2$): 35-45 mmHg
- Partial pressure of oxygen (PaO_2): ≥80 mmHg
- Bicarbonate concentration (HCO_3^-): 22-26 mEq/L
- Oxygen saturation (SaO_2): ≥95%

The relationship between these elements, particularly the $PaCO_2$ and the PaO_2 indicates respiratory status. For example, $PaCO_2$ >55 and the PaO_2 <60 in a patient previously in good health indicates respiratory failure. There are many issues to consider. Ventilator management may require a higher $PaCO_2$ to prevent barotrauma and a lower PaO_2 to reduce oxygen toxicity.

> **Review Video: Blood Gases**
> Visit mometrix.com/academy and enter code: 611909

PULSE OXIMETRY

Pulse oximetry can be initiated by placing a pulse oximeter probe on a thin portion of a patient's anatomy, such as over a fingertip or an earlobe. When connected to a monitor, a light on one end of the probe comes on. It emits red and infrared waves to the other side of the probe. The pulse oximeter then measures the amount of oxygen bound to the hemoglobin, taking into account the fact that hemoglobin with less oxygen bound to it is darker in color than hemoglobin that is replete with oxygen. That measurement is then calculated as the patient's SpO_2.

RELIABILITY OF MONITORING

Care should be taken in monitoring pulse oximetry, as a number of factors can interfere with the accuracy of the results. Decreased arterial flow secondary to hypothermia or hypotension can result in ineffective pulse oximetry. Anemia may cause an inaccurate SpO_2 value, as can hyperlipidemia.

If the patient's venous pressure is elevated, the patient's SpO_2 may be inaccurate. If the patient's SpO_2 is inaccurate and does not match the patient's clinical picture, it may be the result of technical factors, such as motion artifact. Strong ambient light may also cause interference in SpO_2 monitoring.

NURSING INTERVENTIONS

The patient's oxygen saturation should be assessed and charted along with their vital signs. A general respiratory assessment should be completed and the plethysmographic (pleth) waveform should be assessed to ensure that perfusion is adequate. If the pleth is poor, the patient's clinical picture should be further assessed to see if the problem is due to the patient's medical status or arising from equipment difficulties. A poor pleth might be the result of cool extremities, or a loose lead connection. Timely troubleshooting should be undertaken to ensure that all equipment is properly functioning. The pulse oximetry probe placement should be rotated to prevent tissue breakdown, and frequent skin care around the probe should be performed.

CAPNOGRAPHY WITH END-TIDAL CO2 DETECTOR

Capnometry utilizes an **end-tidal CO_2 (ETCO) detector** that measures the concentration of CO_2 in expired air, usually through pH sensitive paper that changes color (commonly purple to yellow). Typically, the capnometer is attached to the ETT and a bag-valve-mask (BVM) ventilator. The capnogram provides data in the shape of a waveform that represents the partial pressure of exhaled gas. It is often used to confirm placement of endotracheal tubes as clinical assessment is not always sufficient, and it is a noninvasive mode of monitoring carbon dioxide in the respiratory cycle. Information provided by the capnogram includes:

- $PaCO_2$ level
- Type and degree of bronchial obstruction, such as COPD (waveform changes from rectangular to a fin-like)
- Air leaks in the ventilation system
- Rebreathing precipitated by need for new CO_2 absorber
- Cardiac arrest
- Hypothermia or reduced metabolism

The normal capnogram is a waveform that represents the varying CO_2 level throughout the breath cycle:

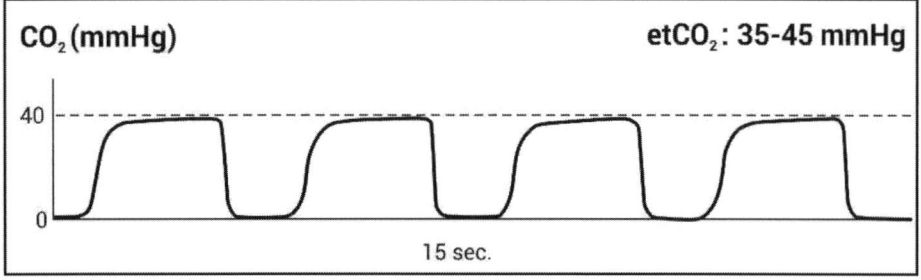

CMC Practice Test

Want to take this practice test in an online interactive format? Check out the online resources page, which includes interactive practice questions and much more: **mometrix.com/resources719/cmc-22549**

1. A 56-year-old woman is monitored in the inpatient telemetry unit. It is noted that she had an episode of non-sustained ventricular tachycardia. The patient was asymptomatic during the episode. What diagnostic test should be performed for further evaluation?

    a. Cardiac computed tomography or magnetic resonance imaging
    b. Transthoracic echocardiography
    c. Angiography
    d. Cardiac enzymes and troponin levels

2. A nurse's patient is being discharged with warfarin as a new medication. The nurse should instruct the patient to avoid which of the following?

    a. Green, leafy vegetables
    b. Rivaroxaban
    c. Multivitamins
    d. Acetaminophen

3. An indirect or estimated value that can be obtained from pulmonary artery catheterization as opposed to a direct measurement is

    a. central venous pressure.
    b. pulmonary artery pressure.
    c. pulmonary vascular resistance.
    d. right-sided intracardiac pressure.

4. A patient with decompensated heart failure is started on an infusion of IV dobutamine in the intensive care unit. The next day, the nurse knows that the medication is effective when she sees which one of the following readings from the patient's pulmonary artery (Swan-Ganz) catheter?

    a. CI: 3 L/min/m^2
    b. CO: 2 L/min
    c. CVP: 15 mmHg
    d. PAOP: 15 mmHg

5. A patient is admitted to the hospital with a newly diagnosed abdominal aortic aneurysm. During assessment, the nurse would expect to auscultate:

    a. a bruit in the central abdomen
    b. hyperactive bowel sounds
    c. muffled heart sounds
    d. a new S4 gallop

6. A 72-year-old man with chronic systolic congestive heart failure is hospitalized due to worsening of his symptoms. He is initially stable, but on the second day of his hospitalization, he suddenly develops chest pain, worsening cough, and rapidly worsening shortness of breath. An electrocardiogram reveals an acute, left-sided, ST-segment elevation myocardial infarction. What is the most likely cause of his shortness of breath?

    a. Pulmonary embolism
    b. Pneumonia
    c. Pulmonary edema
    d. Reactive airway disease

7. The nurse is caring for a 72-year-old man who was admitted to the hospital to rule out acute coronary syndrome. While the nurse is in the room talking to the patient, he suddenly clutches his chest and then falls back on his bed unresponsive. The nurse calls for help and begins cardiopulmonary resuscitation. A team arrives with the crash cart and attaches a monitor/defibrillator to the patient's chest. The monitor reveals asystole. What should the next immediate action be?

    a. Shock the patient.
    b. Resume chest compressions.
    c. Insert an advanced airway.
    d. Give 1 mg of epinephrine intravenously.

8. The nurse is caring for a patient in the ICU 1 hour status post carotid endarterectomy. Which one of the following findings should be the most concerning to the nurse?

    a. High-pitched, musical sound when breathing
    b. Numbness in the neck and shoulder after intraoperative nerve block
    c. Systolic blood pressure of 155 mmHg
    d. Headache pain rated at 5/10

9. A nurse is caring for a patient newly admitted to the critical care unit with diabetic ketoacidosis (DKA). When the patient's basic metabolic panel results return, the nurse would most likely expect to see which one of the following electrolyte imbalances?

    a. Hyperkalemia
    b. Hypokalemia
    c. Hypercalcemia
    d. Hypocalcemia

10. A patient presents to the hospital after experiencing a sudden onset of numbness in the right side of her face and her right arm. She also has drooping of the right side of her mouth and right arm weakness. Computed tomography reveals that the patient has suffered an acute ischemic stroke. When should cardiac monitoring be used in a patient who has had an acute ischemic stroke?

    a. Cardiac monitoring is recommended during the first 24 hours after ischemic stroke onset in all patients.
    b. Cardiac monitoring is not necessary if the patient remains alert and responsive after the stroke.
    c. Cardiac monitoring is only necessary if the electrocardiogram shows abnormalities, such as concomitant acute cardiac ischemia.
    d. Cardiac monitoring is not necessary unless there is high suspicion that a cardiac complication is related to the stroke.

11. A nurse is providing discharge education to a patient with new diagnoses of hyperlipidemia and peripheral arterial disease. The nurse knows that this patient requires additional education when he makes which one of the following comments?

    a. "If I feel pain in my legs while walking, I will pause until the pain subsides."
    b. "If I develop pain in my legs, nonpharmacological options for pain relief include applying ice packs and massage."
    c. "I will plan to take simvastatin at night before bed."
    d. "I understand that I should avoid drinking too much coffee."

12. A patient presents with anxiety, palpitations, tremor, heat intolerance, and weight loss. Laboratory studies reveal that the patient has low thyroid-stimulating hormone and high triiodothyronine (T3) and thyroxine (T4). Which of the following medications would be useful in relieving the patient's palpitations?

    a. Captopril
    b. Hydralazine
    c. Amlodipine
    d. Propranolol

13. When listening to a patient's heart sounds, the nurse notes that the first heart sound is followed by a high-pitched, holosystolic murmur heard best at the apex. The murmur sounds like it is radiating to the patient's axilla. What does this murmur most likely indicate?

    a. Mitral regurgitation
    b. Mitral stenosis
    c. Aortic regurgitation
    d. Aortic stenosis

14. Which of the following is the most specific and sensitive cardiac blood marker for acute myocardial infarction?

    a. Troponin
    b. Creatine kinase–myoglobin
    c. Total creatine kinase
    d. B-type natriuretic peptide

15. A patient in the trauma ICU is in acute renal failure as a result of multiple internal injuries sustained in a motor vehicle crash. The nurse is preparing to start the patient on continuous venovenous hemofiltration (CVVH) dialysis. The nurse understands that all of the following are components of this type of continuous renal replacement therapy EXCEPT:

    a. Dialysate
    b. Replacement fluid
    c. Blood flow
    d. Ultrafiltrate

16. A 68-year-old woman presents with acute substernal chest pain and dyspnea. An electrocardiogram reveals deep T-wave inversion with QT-interval prolongation. Laboratory analysis reveals very mild elevation of troponin and cardiac enzymes. The patient had no history of cardiac disease. Shortly before her symptoms developed, she had been told that her daughter and grandchild had been killed in a car accident. Echocardiography showed left ventricular (LV) apical ballooning with dyskinesis of the apical one-half of the LV. Coronary angiography demonstrated only mild coronary atherosclerosis. When the patient was reevaluated weeks later, it was shown that she had recovered normal LV function. What did this patient most likely experience?

   a. Psychosomatic chest pain
   b. Takotsubo cardiomyopathy
   c. A myocardial infarction
   d. Hypertrophic cardiomyopathy

17. A 28-year-old woman is admitted to the nurse's unit with suspected endocarditis. The patient appears acutely ill, and it is decided that antibiotic therapy should be started as soon as possible. In what manner should blood cultures be obtained in this case?

   a. Obtain one blood culture immediately, then start empiric antibiotic therapy; collect two more blood samples over the next 12–24 hours.
   b. Start empiric antibiotic therapy immediately, and then collect three blood samples as soon as possible.
   c. Obtain three blood cultures over a 1-hour period before beginning empiric antibiotic therapy.
   d. Collect three blood samples over a 24-hour period before beginning empiric antibiotic therapy.

18. A 32-year-old patient in the cardiovascular ICU was admitted 2 weeks ago with a diagnosis of COVID-19 pneumonia and ARDS. The patient was intubated 10 days ago with a #7 endotracheal tube and was placed on venovenous extracorporeal membrane oxygenation 5 days ago. The patient's ventilator settings are as follows:

   Volume Assist Control: 12 breaths per minute
   TV: 420
   FiO_2: 75%
   PEEP: 25

The patient requires vasopressor support, sedation, and pharmacological paralysis. The nurse should anticipate the need to provide education to the family on which one of the following?

   a. Left ventricular assist device (LVAD)
   b. Tracheostomy
   c. Plasmapheresis
   d. Lung transplant

19. A patient on a continuous home infusion of epoprostenol for pulmonary hypertension is hospitalized due to increased exercise intolerance. The provider gives orders to increase the dose of the epoprostenol to address the symptoms. As the dose is titrated up, the nurse knows to closely monitor the patient for:

   a. bronchospasm
   b. sudden hearing loss
   c. nausea and vomiting
   d. hypertension

20. A patient with a history of Addison's disease was admitted complaining of extreme fatigue for the past several days, new flank pain and nausea, and new generalized weakness. The nurse notes hyperpigmentation in the patient's face and hands. The patient's vital signs are:

   HR: 88 and regular
   BP: 85/52 mmHg
   O_2 sat: 96%
   Temp: 97.8 °F
   RR: 20

What order does the nurse anticipate receiving from the provider first?

   a. Inject 100 mg hydrocortisone via IV one time stat.
   b. Insert a nasogastric tube and set it to intermittent suction.
   c. Prepare the patient for an abdominal computed tomography scan.
   d. Collect a urine sample for urine analysis and culture via clean catch.

21. The nurse is caring for a patient in the ICU with a diagnosis of dilated cardiomyopathy. The patient's ejection fraction is 10% based on the results of the transthoracic echocardiogram, and the central venous pressure reading is 24 with jugular venous distension present upon assessment. The patient is in atrial fibrillation with a heart rate of 80–110 bpm. Which one of the following orders should the nurse question?

   a. Furosemide 40 mg IVP two times a day
   b. Amiodarone 400 mg PO two times a day
   c. Warfarin 5 mg PO daily
   d. Verapamil 80 mg PO three times a day

22. A patient in the ICU is receiving continuous renal replacement therapy. The machine's high-venous-pressure alarm is sounding. What is the most likely cause of this alarm?

   a. Low blood pressure
   b. Clotting in the line
   c. Air bubbles in the line
   d. Too much fluid removal

23. A patient admitted to the ICU following a transcatheter aortic valve replacement has a hematoma to the incision site that has increased in size since admission. The patient rates sudden back pain at 8 out of 10, and the patient's blood pressure is 85/42 mmHg. Which one of the following orders should the nurse implement first?

   a. Administer 1 liter bolus of 0.9% sodium chloride.
   b. Start norepinephrine infusion to maintain a MAP goal of >65.
   c. Collect a stat complete blood count.
   d. Administer hydromorphone 0.5 mg IV push (IVP) stat.

24. An 81-year-old woman is on her third day of hospitalization for an exacerbation of her chronic congestive heart failure. Her symptoms have improved over the course of her stay. The nurse notes that her vital signs are as follows:

   HR: 90
   BP: 131/88 mmHg
   O₂ sat: 81% on room air
   RR: 18

Her SaO₂ on room air for the past day has been over 95%. She appears to be breathing comfortably at this time and does not appear ill. What is the first thing that the nurse should do?

   a. Place the patient on 100% oxygen by nasal cannula.
   b. Place the patient on 100% oxygen by non-rebreather mask.
   c. Recheck the patient's pulse oximetry.
   d. Page the patient's physician immediately.

25. A typical presentation of a patient with unstable angina is best described as chest discomfort or pain that is

   a. difficult to describe, begins at rest, and lasts for longer than 20 minutes.
   b. described as sharp and stabbing and improves when the patient is sitting up or leaning forward.
   c. difficult to describe, begins while the patient is exercising, and resolves within 2–5 minutes after resting.
   d. described as sharp and is reproducible on examination.

26. A 47-year-old woman presents to the hospital with a blood pressure of 220/130 mmHg. She is confused and restless on arrival and is unable to answer questions. Her family reports that she complained of a bad headache and nausea earlier in the day. Her husband notes that she stopped taking her blood pressure medications over the past few days because she did not feel like she needed them anymore. What is the most appropriate treatment approach?

   a. Slowly lower the patient's systolic blood pressure to 120 mmHg with intravenous (IV) antihypertensive medication, and then switch to oral antihypertensive medication for maintenance.
   b. Slowly lower the patient's diastolic blood pressure to 85 mmHg with oral antihypertensive medication, and then adjust the dose of antihypertensive medication to maintain blood pressure.
   c. Rapidly lower the patient's systolic blood pressure to 120 mmHg with oral antihypertensive medication, and then adjust the dose of antihypertensive medication to maintain blood pressure.
   d. Rapidly lower the patient's diastolic blood pressure to 100 mmHg with IV antihypertensive medication, and then gradually reduce the diastolic pressure to 85 mmHg with oral antihypertensive medication.

27. If a patient has already received fibrinolytic therapy for an acute ST-segment elevation myocardial infarction, when is additional treatment with percutaneous coronary intervention (PCI) most likely to be recommended?

    a. If possible, all patients should receive PCI 2 hours after receiving fibrinolytic therapy.
    b. Patients who have hemodynamic instability, despite fibrinolytic therapy, should receive PCI.
    c. Stable patients who have been found to have an occluded infarct-related artery should receive PCI.
    d. If the fibrinolytic therapy was given within the past 2 hours, the patient should receive PCI.

28. During what time period should a patient be monitored for heparin-induced thrombocytopenia after starting heparin therapy?

    a. Over the first 5–10 days after initiating therapy
    b. Over the first 3–4 weeks after initiating therapy
    c. After the patient has been on therapy for over 2 weeks
    d. After the patient has been on therapy for over 1 month

29. The nurse is caring for a 62-year-old patient in the ICU status post carotid endarterectomy. The patient has a history of chronic obstructive pulmonary disease (COPD), diabetes mellitus type 2, and congestive heart failure. The patient's vital signs are as follows:

    HR: 58
    BP: 175/99 mmHg
    O_2 sat: 93% 2L by nasal cannula
    Temp: 99 °F

The nurse should take which action next?

    a. Increase the patient's oxygen to 4 L by nasal cannula.
    b. Administer labetalol 20 mg IVP.
    c. Administer hydralazine 10 mg IVP.
    d. Administer acetaminophen 650 mg by mouth.

30. What life-threatening arrhythmia is associated with the long QT syndrome?

    a. Wolff-Parkinson-White syndrome
    b. Sick sinus syndrome
    c. Torsade de pointes
    d. Ventricular fibrillation

31. What is the recommended length of time between initial medical contact and primary percutaneous coronary intervention in a patient with an ST-segment elevation myocardial infarction ("door-to-balloon" time)?

    a. 30 minutes
    b. 90 minutes
    c. 2 hours
    d. 4 hours

32. A patient has been admitted to the ICU following a syncopal episode. The patient is short of breath, requiring oxygen at 4L by nasal cannula; his blood pressure is 88/45 mmHg; and he has the following electrocardiogram rhythm:

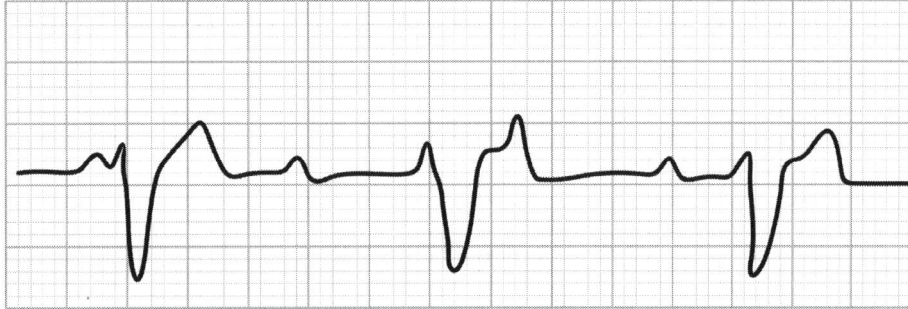

Which one of the following treatments is most appropriate for this patient?

    a. Atropine 1 mg IVP
    b. Amiodarone 150 mg IVP
    c. Transcutaneous pacing
    d. Cardioversion

33. A patient with a history of congestive heart failure presents with dyspnea, cough, and peripheral edema. On physical examination, the patient is found to be hypotensive with diminished distal pulses. Crackles in the lungs and chest x-ray findings indicate the presence of pulmonary congestion. Laboratory testing reveals that renal insufficiency is also present. What initial treatment should the nurse give the patient?

    a. Loop diuretics
    b. Thiazide diuretics
    c. Angiotensin-converting enzyme inhibitors
    d. Inotropes

34. A patient has been transferred to the ICU after a transcatheter aortic valve replacement (TAVR) via the transfemoral route. The patient is alert and oriented ×4, and his family is at the bedside. The nurse is providing postprocedure instructions to the patient. What information should the nurse include?

    a. The patient will need to take clopidogrel for the rest of his life.
    b. The patient's daily aspirin dose is no longer needed.
    c. The patient will need to lie flat for 6 hours.
    d. The patient's left arm should not be lifted higher than his shoulder for 1 week.

35. Which of the following arterial blood gas values is abnormal?

    a. pH: 7.38
    b. PCO_2: 43 mmHg
    c. PaO_2: 99 mmHg
    d. HCO_3: 14 mEq/L

36. A patient is in the critical care unit due to an acute ischemic stroke with an onset of symptoms 12 hours earlier. The patient is not a candidate for thrombolysis due to a recent surgery. The nurse would expect to monitor the patient's blood pressure closely and keep it in compliance with which of the following criteria?

    a. Less than 250/150 mmHg
    b. Less than 220/120 mmHg
    c. Less than 180/95 mmHg
    d. Between 90/60 and 120/80 mmHg

37. A nurse is caring for a patient who just received arterial bypass surgery to the lower right leg due to peripheral artery disease. Four hours after the procedure, the nurse notes a decreased pedal pulse and new dusky coloration of the right foot. The patient reports numbness in the right foot. What does the nurse anticipate is likely happening?

    a. Graft failure
    b. Peripheral nerve damage
    c. Deep vein thrombosis
    d. Compartment syndrome

38. A faint heart murmur that can be heard only when concentrating is most likely what grade?

    a. Grade I
    b. Grade II
    c. Grade III
    d. Grade IV

39. A 19-year-old patient presents with the sudden onset of chest pain and dyspnea. His vital signs are as follows:

    HR: 110
    BP: 100/60 mmHg
    O_2 sat: 88%
    RR: 30

Physical examination reveals diminished breath sounds on the left side. Chest radiograph reveals a hyperlucent line along the left chest wall. All of the following are risk factors associated with this patient's condition EXCEPT

    a. hypertension.
    b. gender.
    c. mechanical ventilation.
    d. smoking.

40. A patient reports shortness of breath and sternum pain that radiates down the left arm. The patient's troponin levels are elevated. The heart rhythm is sinus tachycardia, and the electrocardiogram appears normal within all leads. The patient has no history of cardiac dysfunction or similar episodes. Which one of the following orders would NOT be appropriate?

    a. Adminsiter0.3 mg of nitroglycerin sublingually.
    b. Prepare the patient for cardiac catheterization within 90 minutes.
    c. Administer 325 mg of aspirin orally.
    d. Insert a 16-gauge IV catheter.

41. A nurse is caring for a patient with acute respiratory distress syndrome who is intubated in the intensive care unit. The patient is being kept sedated with benzodiazepines at this time. In addition to improving tolerance of mechanical ventilation, sedation is specifically useful in this patient for which of the following reasons?

    a. It will improve blood flow.
    b. It acts as an analgesic.
    c. It decreases glucose consumption.
    d. It decreases oxygen consumption.

42. A 30-year-old woman complains of chest pain and palpitations and is subsequently diagnosed with pericarditis. An echocardiogram reveals signs of a pericardial effusion. Vital signs are as follows:

    HR: 94
    BP: 117/68 mmHg
    O_2 sat: 100% on room air
    Temp: 98.5 °F
    RR: 15

The patient has no significant medical history. What is the most appropriate way to proceed at this time?

    a. Schedule a pericardiocentesis to drain the pericardial fluid, and treat the underlying condition.
    b. Treat the underlying condition, but do not drain the effusion.
    c. Schedule a surgical pericardiectomy to drain the effusion, and treat the underlying condition.
    d. Monitor the patient with telemetry until the effusion resolves.

43. A nurse is caring for a patient undergoing continuous renal replacement therapy. The nurse knows to monitor the patient closely for which one of the following complications?

    a. Hypothermia
    b. Pulmonary edema
    c. pruritus
    d. Hypertension

44. Which one of the following medications reduces dysrhythmias by blocking calcium channels in the cells of the myocardium?

    a. Amiodarone
    b. Propranolol
    c. Lidocaine
    d. Diltiazem

45. A patient presents with chest pain, severe hypotension, tachycardia, agitation, and cool, clammy skin. Lung examination reveals diffuse crackles. Other physical examination findings include diminished distal arterial pulses and increased jugular venous pressure. Which of the following combination of signs and symptoms makes cardiogenic shock a more likely diagnosis than hypovolemic or distributive shock?

    a. Diffuse crackles in the lungs and increased jugular venous pressure
    b. Chest pain and tachycardia
    c. Diminished distal arterial pulses and cool, clammy skin
    d. Severe hypotension and agitation

46. Major mechanical complications of acute myocardial infarction include all of the following EXCEPT

a. rupture of the left ventricular free wall.
b. rupture of the interventricular septum.
c. the development of mitral regurgitation.
d. the development of aortic regurgitation.

47. A patient in the ICU has received a left ventricular assist device (LVAD) for end-stage heart failure. The nurse should ensure adequate fluid intake to prevent which one of the following complications that can result from hypovolemia?

a. Infection
b. Hypertension
c. Suction event
d. Pump thrombus

48. When should transesophageal echocardiography be the initial test of choice as opposed to transthoracic echocardiography?

a. With suspected pericardial effusion
b. To evaluate left ventricle ejection fraction
c. With suspected cardiomyopathy
d. With suspected acute aortic dissection

49. A patient is in the critical care unit due to infective endocarditis. The patient develops increased anxiety and shortness of breath over the course of a couple hours. The nurse notes new muffled heart sounds and new jugular venous distension. The patient's lung sounds are clear. The nurse observes the patient's arterial line reading and notes that the blood pressure drops whenever the patient inhales. The nurse zeroes the arterial line and ensures accurate readings. The waveform is appropriate. The patient's readings include:

HR: 120 bpm
Systolic BP: fluctuating between 80 and 95 mmHg
Diastolic BP: fluctuating between 65 and 70 mmHg
Pulse pressure: 20–25 mmHg

What does the nurse anticipate the patient is experiencing?

a. Acute congestive heart failure exacerbation
b. Mitral valve prolapse
c. Tension pneumothorax
d. Cardiac tamponade

50. The nurse in the ICU is caring for an intubated patient. Sedation has been discontinued in preparation for the daily spontaneous breathing trial. The patient is awake and alert and is following commands. The patient's vitals are as follows:

> RR: 22
> O2 sat: 98% on ventilator, ventilator settings:
> > Volume Assist Control: 12 breaths per minute
> > TV: 450
> > PEEP: 5
> > Pressure Support: 5

Which one of the following actions should the nurse include in the patient's plan of care to prevent ventilator-acquired pneumonia?

 a. Provide incentive spirometry sessions every hour while awake.
 b. Change ventilator circuits every shift.
 c. Perform intermittent subglottic suctioning as tolerated.
 d. Turn/reposition the patient every 2 hours.

51. Which of the following patients would be eligible for an exercise electrocardiogram stress test?

 a. An active 65-year-old woman with a right bundle branch block
 b. An active 68-year-old woman who has a paced ventricular rhythm
 c. An active 62-year-old man with a left bundle branch block
 d. An active 60-year-old man with Wolff-Parkinson-White syndrome

52. A nurse is providing discharge education to a patient who just received a new implantable cardioverter defibrillator. The nurse knows that the patient requires correction when the patient makes which one of the following comments?

 a. "I will not lift my arm above my shoulder for the rest of the day."
 b. "I will not carry my grandson for the next 2 weeks."
 c. "I will no longer be able to swim or take a bath."
 d. "If I receive a shock and am not feeling well, I should call 911 right away."

53. A patient has been admitted to the ICU for targeted temperature management after a myocardial infarction and cardiac arrest. The nurse should expect all of the following orders EXCEPT:

 a. At 24 hr of hypothermia, begin to rewarm the patient at 2 °C/hr.
 b. Monitor the patient's temperature continuously using bladder or esophageal temperature monitoring.
 c. Cool the patient as quickly as possible to 32 °C.
 d. Administer a cisatracurium bolus and continuous infusion.

54. ST-segment elevation that is seen diffusely in most or all limb and precordial leads is most likely indicative of

 a. acute myocardial infarction.
 b. cardiac tamponade.
 c. pericarditis.
 d. left ventricular hypertrophy.

55. A patient returns to the critical care unit after undergoing a transradial cardiac catheterization. In order to assess for adequate blood flow through the radial artery, the nurse would complete which one of the following assessments?

    a. Palmar grasp test
    b. Brachioradialis reflex test
    c. Barbeau test
    d. Reverse Barbeau test

56. Permanent cardiac pacing is a beneficial option with all of the following clinical conditions EXCEPT

    a. symptomatic sinus bradycardia.
    b. torsade de pointes associated with hypokalemia.
    c. second-degree atrioventricular Mobitz II block.
    d. significant carotid sinus hypersensitivity.

57. A nurse is caring for a patient following an MI. The patient develops increased confusion over the course of the morning. The nurse notes fine crackles throughout both lungs on auscultation, and the patient has a frequent productive cough with pink frothy sputum. The patient's vital signs are:

    HR: 95 and regular
    BP: 94/58 mmHg
    O_2 sat: 86% on nasal cannula 2 LPM
    Temp: 98.4 °F
    RR: 26

What order does the nurse anticipate from the provider?

    a. Administer ceftriaxone 2 g via IV.
    b. Prepare the patient for chest tube insertion.
    c. Administer furosemide 40 mg via IV.
    d. Prepare the patient for intubation and mechanical ventilation.

58. A nurse is caring for a patient on the telemetry unit who was admitted following a syncopal episode at home. The patient has presented as alert and oriented and has been hemodynamically stable throughout his hospitalization. The nurse suddenly observes that the patient has become unresponsive. His pulse is palpable. His vital signs are now:

> HR: 156 and irregular
> BP: 78/36 mmHg
> O₂ sat: 90%
> Temp: 97.5 °F
> RR: 28

The nurse also notes the following rhythm on the telemetry monitor:

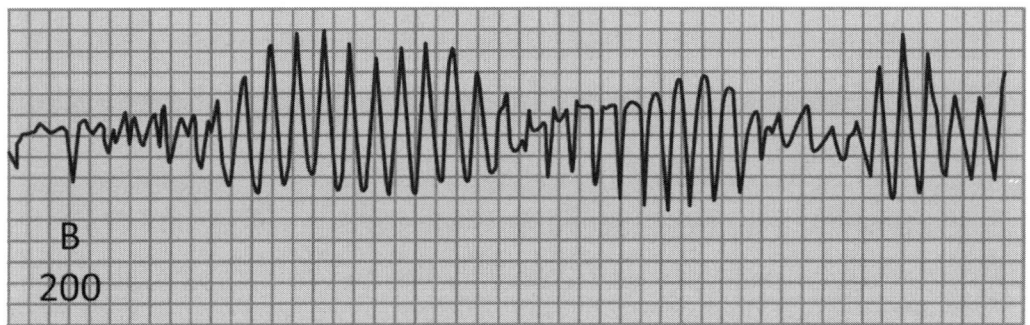

The nurse should anticipate and prepare for which one of the following orders?

a. Defibrillate and inject magnesium sulfate 2 g IV.
b. Defibrillate and inject epinephrine 1 mg IV.
c. Prepare for cardioversion and inject magnesium sulfate 2 g IV.
d. Prepare for cardioversion and inject amiodarone 300 mg IV.

59. A 34-year-old man is brought to the emergency department because of chest pain. It is quickly determined that he is experiencing an acute ST-segment elevation myocardial infarction as a result of cocaine ingestion. How should this patient's initial treatment differ from other instances of acute coronary syndrome?

a. Aspirin use should be avoided in the acute setting.
b. Beta-blocker use should be avoided in the acute setting.
c. Supplemental oxygen use is not necessary in the acute setting.
d. Nitroglycerin use should be avoided in the acute setting.

60. A patient in the ICU is intubated and receiving inhaled nitric oxide for severe pulmonary hypertension. The nurse will need to monitor the patient for which one of the following adverse effects of nitric oxide administration?

a. Hypercapnia
b. Oxygen toxicity
c. Methemoglobinemia
d. Volume overload

61. The nurse is caring for a patient in the ICU with stage IV pulmonary hypertension. The nurse recognizes that the primary action of inhaled nitric oxide therapy is to:

    a. Reduce fluid overload
    b. Reduce serum bicarbonate
    c. Dilate the pulmonary vessels
    d. Prevent a pulmonary embolus

62. A patient diagnosed with influenza is in the ICU with a diagnosis of ARDS. The patient is intubated and sedated on propofol and fentanyl. The ventilator is set at assist control with a rate of 22 breaths per minute, tidal volume of 4 mL/kg, PEEP of 20, and FiO2 of 75%. The patient is on continuous vasopressin and a norepinephrine drip. The patient's vitals are as follows:

    Heart rate: 122
    Temperature: 100.9 °F
    Blood pressure: 109/58 mmHg
    Oxygen saturation: 93%

The patient's chest x-ray shows interstitial edema and perihilar opacities. The nurse should anticipate all of the following orders EXCEPT?

    a. Give a 0.9% sodium chloride bolus of 30 cc/kg.
    b. Prone the patient 16 hr, then supine 8 hr/day.
    c. Initiate tube feedings at 20 mL/hr.
    d. Maintain plateau pressure <30 cmH$_2$O.

63. Two days after having an ST-elevation myocardial infarction (STEMI), a patient notifies the nurse of stabbing pain in the left sternal region, but some relief occurs when the head of the bed is elevated upright. The nurse auscultates a scratch-like murmur with each heartbeat. A 12-lead electrocardiogram shows ST elevation in all leads. The nurse notifies the physician and anticipates receiving which one of the following orders first?

    a. Give nitroglycerin 0.3 mg sublingual stat.
    b. Prepare the patient for emergent cardiac catheterization.
    c. Give ibuprofen 800 mg now and every 8 hours thereafter.
    d. Give intravenous (IV) morphine sulfate 2 mg as needed for pain.

64. A patient is newly admitted to the critical care unit for treatment of acute respiratory distress syndrome. The patient is intubated and mechanically ventilated with an initial positive end-expiratory pressure (PEEP) setting of 8 and a fraction of inspired oxygen (FiO$_2$) setting of 30% with plans to titrate these settings based on the patient's status. The patient's current oxygen saturation is 82%. The nurse anticipates which one of the following vent changes of the PEEP and FiO$_2$ settings?

    a. Increasing the PEEP to 10 and maintaining the FiO$_2$ at 30%
    b. Increasing the PEEP to 10 and increasing the FiO$_2$ to 50%
    c. Increasing the FiO$_2$ to 80% and maintaining the PEEP at 8
    d. Increasing the FiO$_2$ to 100% and decreasing the PEEP to 5

65. A 72-year-old man complains of chest pain, shortness of breath, and dizziness. His vital signs are as follows:

HR: 120
BP: 78/50 mmHg
O₂ sat: 95%
RR: 20

His blood pressure 1 hour before this was 122/75 mmHg. His electrocardiogram is normal other than the presence of tachycardia. What action should be taken first?

a. Draw arterial blood gases.
b. Begin giving the patient 100% oxygen through a nasal cannula.
c. Give the patient a low dose of nitroglycerin while monitoring blood pressure.
d. Establish intravenous access immediately with a large-bore intravenous catheter.

66. Which of the following medications has been shown to play a role in preventing congestive heart failure?

a. Calcium channel blockers
b. Angiotensin-converting enzyme inhibitors
c. Anticoagulants
d. Loop diuretics

67. A patient presents with chest pain, elevated jugular venous pressure, cyanosis, a right ventricular heave, and sinus tachycardia on electrocardiogram. He has been bedridden for the past week following surgery. Vital signs are as follows:

HR: 115
BP: 100/60 mmHg
O₂ sat: 80% on room air
RR: 40

The patient remains persistently hypotensive. Which of the following should be done first?

a. Ventilation/perfusion scan
b. Computed tomography pulmonary angiogram
c. Administration of tissue-type plasminogen activator (tPA)
d. Administration of warfarin

68. A routine x-ray shows that a patient has an asymptomatic descending thoracic aortic aneurysm. The aneurysm has a diameter of 4 cm. What is the recommended initial management?

a. Beta-blockers for aggressive blood pressure control and surveillance
b. Surveillance only
c. Surgical correction
d. Aspirin, aggressive blood pressure control with a beta-blocker, an angiotensin-converting enzyme inhibitor, and surveillance

69. A patient has been admitted to the ICU after being found unresponsive at home. Upon arrival at the ICU, the patient becomes unresponsive again, and goes into ventricular fibrillation. Cardiopulmonary resuscitation (CPR) is initiated, and a return of spontaneous circulation is obtained. The team inserts a Swan-Ganz catheter and an arterial line. Initial readings reveal the following:

> Blood pressure: 88/44 mmHg
> Mean arterial pressure (MAP): 58
> Central venous pressure: 22
> Cardiac index: 1.8
> Cardiac output: 2.5
> Pulmonary arterial wedge pressure: 52

Which one of the following orders should the nurse question?

a. Dobutamine infusion at 2 mcg/kg/min
b. Normal saline 1 L bolus
c. Norepinephrine infusion to maintain the mean arterial pressure at >65
d. Furosemide 40 mg intravenous push (IVP) stat

70. **Binge drinking puts patients at significantly higher risk for which cardiac dysrhythmia?**

a. Atrial fibrillation
b. Ventricular fibrillation
c. Bradycardia
d. Premature ventricular contractions

71. **A patient complains of right-sided calf pain. The nurse decides to evaluate the patient for a possible deep venous thrombosis (DVT). All of the following signs or symptoms are typical of a DVT EXCEPT**

a. unilateral swelling of the calf.
b. warmth.
c. skin breakdown.
d. superficial venous dilation.

72. **A patient being monitored on telemetry suddenly develops a completely erratic rhythm on the monitor with no distinguishable waves. When the nurse comes into the room, the patient is unarousable. What dysrhythmia is likely to be the cause?**

a. Atrial flutter
b. Atrial fibrillation
c. Ventricular flutter
d. Ventricular fibrillation

73. **A patient presents to the hospital with atrial fibrillation. It is unknown how long the patient has been in atrial fibrillation. The patient did not convert to a regular sinus rhythm with medical treatment, so it is decided to continue the patient on medication for rate control and anticoagulation. It is also decided that cardioversion should be attempted. Ideally cardioversion should be attempted**

a. immediately to eradicate the arrhythmia.
b. after the patient has had 3–5 days of anticoagulation.
c. after the patient has had 3–4 weeks of anticoagulation.
d. after the patient has had 3–4 months of anticoagulation.

74. A patient presents with cardiogenic shock following an acute myocardial infarction (MI). How should this patient's treatment differ from that of acute MI without shock?

a. Lidocaine should be used in higher doses than usual.
b. Calcium channel blockers should be avoided.
c. Clopidogrel should be given before angiography.
d. Aspirin therapy should be avoided.

75. A patient presents with palpitations, dizziness, nausea, and chest discomfort. The patient is quickly placed on a cardiac monitor, which reveals a polymorphic ventricular tachycardia that is identified as torsade de pointes. Which of the following electrolyte imbalances is a risk factor for developing torsade de pointes?

a. Hypercalcemia
b. Hypomagnesemia
c. Hyperkalemia
d. Hypochloremia

76. A patient is in the critical care unit following an MI and subsequent cardiogenic shock. An intra-aortic balloon pump (IABP) with 1:1 support has been in place for 24 hours. A new echocardiogram shows a left ventricular ejection fraction value of 40%. The patient's current vital signs are:

HR: 90 and regular
BP: 95/62 mmHg
CI: 2.5 L/min/m²
CVP: 9 mmHg

The nurse anticipates which one of the following orders from the provider?

a. Keep the IABP in place at the current support mode for another 24 hours and then repeat the echocardiogram.
b. Prepare to wean the patient's IABP support from 1:1 to 1:2.
c. Prepare to explant the IABP.
d. Increase the support mode of the IABP.

77. A contraindication for continuous positive airway pressure (CPAP) is when a patient has signs and symptoms of

a. cardiogenic pulmonary edema.
b. a pneumothorax.
c. pneumonia.
d. chronic obstructive pulmonary disease.

78. What is the most serious acute complication associated with coronary artery stenting?

a. Stent fracture
b. Stroke
c. Myocardial infarction
d. Renal failure

79. A patient with end-stage heart failure and a prognosis of less than 6 months to live is experiencing increased activity intolerance, tachypnea, shortness of breath, and chronic congested cough. At discharge to home per the patient's wishes, he is prescribed oral morphine 5 mg every 4 hours as needed. He asks the nurse why he would want this medication if he is not having any pain. Which one of the following is the best response?

   a. "The morphine should be taken to prevent any pain from developing in the future."
   b. "The morphine will decrease your chest congestion."
   c. "The morphine will ease your work of breathing."
   d. "This must have been ordered by mistake. I'll ask the doctor to remove it."

80. Cor pulmonale is a common complication of what disease state?

   a. Chronic atrial fibrillation
   b. Pulmonary hypertension
   c. Pneumonia
   d. Coronary artery disease

81. A 22-year-old patient with Duchenne muscular dystrophy who is in acute respiratory distress is admitted to the ICU from the emergency department. The patient is intubated with the following ventilator settings:

   Volume Assist Control: 12 breaths per minute
   TV: 420
   FiO_2: 60%
   PEEP: 5

The patient has the following arterial blood gas results:

   pH: 7.28
   $PaCO_2$: 59
   HCO_3: 25
   PaO_2: 81

Which one of the following ventilator changes would the nurse anticipate?

   a. Increase the FiO_2.
   b. Reduce the set rate of breaths per minute.
   c. Increase the set rate of breaths per minute.
   d. Increase the PEEP.

82. Several hours after undergoing a cardiac catheterization procedure a patient complains of severe, diffuse, abdominal pain. He then has an episode of bloody diarrhea. What does the nurse suspect may be the cause of his symptoms?

   a. Mesenteric ischemia
   b. Cholecystitis
   c. Acute renal failure
   d. Gastric ulceration

83. A patient is being discharged from the hospital with a new diagnosis of atrial fibrillation. He has started warfarin for anticoagulation. What should the target range of his international normalized ratio be?

   a. 1–2
   b. 1.5–2.5
   c. 2–3
   d. 3–4

84. A 77-year-old patient complains of chest discomfort and seems confused as compared to baseline. A quick check of the vital signs reveals the following:

HR: 44
BP: 86/49 mmHg
O_2 sat: 89%
RR: 18

His pulse is palpable. He is placed on oxygen by nasal cannula, intravenous (IV) access is obtained, and a cardiac monitor/defibrillator is attached. What should the next step in this patient's care?

 a. Begin transcutaneous pacing.
 b. Administer dopamine, 2–10 mcg/min IV.
 c. Administer a 1 mg atropine bolus IV.
 d. Administer epinephrine, 2–10 mcg/min IV.

85. A patient is brought to the hospital after experiencing cardiac arrest. He was resuscitated in the field but did not regain consciousness and then brought to the hospital for further treatment. The targeted temperature management (TTM) protocol is quickly instituted for the patient. The aim of TTM after a cardiac arrest is to prevent

 a. neurological injury.
 b. pulmonary injury.
 c. renal failure.
 d. a stroke.

86. An electrocardiogram (ECG) performed on a patient on the telemetry floor reveals variable PR intervals, a fast atrial rate, and a slow ventricular rate. The atrial beats and ventricular beats do not appear to be related. This patient is likely to have which type of atrioventricular (AV) block listed below?

 a. First-degree AV block
 b. Second-degree AV Mobitz I block
 c. Second-degree AV Mobitz II block
 d. Third-degree AV block

87. A nurse is reviewing discharge orders with a patient who has received a new left ventricular assist device (LVAD) during his hospitalization. The nurse knows that the patient requires further education when he makes which one of the following comments?

 a. "When I'm at home, I will be responsible for changing the driveline dressing myself."
 b. "I should avoid blood-thinning medications due to the risk for bleeding from the driveline site."
 c. "I will run a self-test on my LVAD on a daily basis and notify my provider if there are any warning messages."
 d. "I will drink sufficient fluids to ensure proper blood volume levels."

88. A patient presents with complaints of dyspnea, a feeling of chest fullness, and fatigue. On physical examination, the patient is found to have elevated jugular venous pressure, hypotension, pulsus paradoxus, and tachycardia. An electrocardiogram shows sinus tachycardia, low voltage, and beat-to-beat alterations in the QRS complexes. What is the most likely diagnosis?

 a. Acute myocardial infarction
 b. Pulmonary embolus
 c. Aortic dissection
 d. Cardiac tamponade

89. A patient in the ICU has a diagnosis of dilated cardiomyopathy and has an Impella device in place. The nurse understands that which one of the following is correct regarding the Impella device and cardiopulmonary resuscitation?

 a. Reduce the P-level to P-2 during CPR.
 b. Defibrillation is contraindicated.
 c. CPR should be initiated because the arterial line waveform is flat.
 d. The Impella device must be turned off.

90. A patient in the ICU is 3 days status post ischemic stroke with residual right-sided weakness, right-sided facial droop, and dysphagia. The patient has been evaluated by a speech therapist and has been prescribed a mechanical soft diet with thickened liquids. Which one of the following interventions should the nurse include in the plan of care?

 a. Serve all liquids cold with ice.
 b. Serve sticky foods such as peanut butter whenever possible.
 c. Ensure that the patient uses a straw when drinking.
 d. Avoid giving solids and liquids at the same time.

Answer Key and Explanations

1. B: Asymptomatic non-sustained ventricular tachycardia is often benign, but it is important to rule out any associated structural heart disease. In asymptomatic patients, the initial evaluation should include a thorough history and physical examination, a 12-lead electrocardiogram, transthoracic echocardiography, and exercise stress testing.

2. B: Rivaroxaban is an anticoagulant that can greatly increase bleeding risk if taken concurrently with warfarin. Green, leafy vegetables and multivitamins contain vitamin K, which will decrease the effectiveness of warfarin; however, warfarin dosing can be adjusted accordingly. Patients should be educated about the importance of being consistent with their vitamin K intake so as not to alter their drug effectiveness. Acetaminophen can be taken safely with warfarin.

3. C: Pulmonary vascular resistance, systemic vascular resistance, pulmonary artery wedge pressure, and cardiac output can all be estimated from measurements obtained from pulmonary artery catheterization. Pulmonary artery catheters can directly measure central venous pressure, right-sided intracardiac pressure, and pulmonary arterial pressure.

4. A: The patient's cardiac index (CI) is within the normal range (2.5–4 L/min/m²), which is the goal when starting dobutamine for patients with decompensated heart failure. The patient's cardiac output (CO) is below normal (4–8 L/min), indicating inadequate output from the heart. The patient's central venous pressure (CVP) is also elevated compared to the normal range (8–12 mmHg), which indicates fluid volume overload. The pulmonary artery occlusion pressure (PAOP) is elevated compared to the normal range (4–12 mmHg), which could indicate left ventricular failure or stenosis of the mitral valve.

5. A: An abdominal aortic aneurysm can often produce a whooshing sound, or a bruit, on auscultation of the aorta as the blood rushes through the enlarged vessel. The other sounds listed would not be related to this condition.

6. C: The medical history of the patient described in the question is key to discovering the most likely cause of his shortness of breath. He already had a history of congestive heart failure, which likely developed into acute decompensated heart failure (ADHF) due to his ST-segment elevation myocardial infarction. The ADHF is a fairly common cause of acute respiratory distress and is associated with the rapid accumulation of fluid in the lungs (pulmonary edema). Although a pulmonary embolism, pneumonia, and reactive airway disease may all cause dyspnea, cough, and chest pain, they are less likely in this case due to the patient's history.

7. B: Asystole is not a rhythm that can be shocked (defibrillated) into regularity. One of the most important parts of advanced cardiac life support is to minimize interruptions in chest compressions. In this case, chest compressions should be resumed immediately while the rest of the team prepares for next steps. A team member should ensure that the patient has good intravenous access and 1 mg of epinephrine can be given every 3–5 minutes, but chest compressions should continue while this is taking place. The patient may need to have an advanced airway placed, but once again, chest compressions should be continued while preparations are made.

8. A: The high-pitched, musical breathing sound describes stridor, which is indicative of narrowing of the airway. This must be treated emergently in patients that are post endarterectomy because it indicates swelling that could occlude the airway. The nerve block would not be expected to wear off for at least 6 hours; therefore, numbness is expected. The blood pressure is elevated, but it does not require emergent intervention. A headache of 5/10 severity can occur and should be treated with acetaminophen. If pain medication is not effective in treating the headache, then the physician should be notified.

9. A: Moderate hyperkalemia is commonly seen with patients in DKA. A decrease in circulating insulin leads to an electrolyte shift that causes potassium to leave the cells and enter the bloodstream, thus resulting in elevated levels of serum potassium. DKA does not routinely lead to large shifts in calcium levels; therefore, an excess or deficits of calcium are not something the nurse should expect to see in the patient's bloodwork.

10. A: Cardiac monitoring is recommended for all patients during the first 24 hours after the initial onset of an ischemic stroke. Cardiac monitoring is used to detect atrial fibrillation or other cardiac arrhythmias that may need to be addressed. Atrial fibrillation may suggest cardiac emboli as a possible cause of the stroke. Even if a patient is alert, does not have acute electrocardiographic abnormalities, and does not have a history of cardiac disease, it is important to monitor for cardiac arrhythmias after a stroke.

11. B: Many patients with peripheral arterial disease have underlying hyperlipidemia and plaque buildup in their arteries that leads to decreased circulation. Nurses should educate patients to avoid any actions that would further restrict blood flow, such as applying ice packs. Patients with peripheral arterial disease are also at risk for blood clots, so the nurse should educate the patient to never massage their legs, which can dislodge a clot and result in an embolism. The other comments made by the patient are correct. The patient should be encouraged to get moderate exercise, such as walking, and can pause until any pain resides if they develop claudication. Simvastatin, a cholesterol-lowering medication, is frequently prescribed for hyperlipidemia and is most effective when taken in the evening. The patient should limit his caffeine intake due to the vasoconstrictive effects of caffeine.

12. D: Beta-blockers, such as propranolol and atenolol, are useful in relieving palpitations and slowing the heart rate in patients with hyperthyroidism. Beta-blockers, however, do not treat the underlying cause of these symptoms.

13. A: The murmur of mitral regurgitation may vary, but in its typical presentation, it is holosystolic, begins immediately after S1, is heard best over the apex, and may radiate to the axilla or back. Mitral valve stenosis has a rumbling, mid-diastolic murmur and is heard best with the bell of the stethoscope over the left ventricular impulse. Aortic regurgitation is heard as a blowing, early diastolic murmur that radiates toward the cardiac apex and is often heard best along the left sternal border. Aortic valve stenosis causes a mid-systolic murmur that is typically loudest in the right second intercostal space and may radiate to the carotids.

14. A: Troponin is the preferred cardiac marker for diagnosing acute myocardial infarction (MI) because it has increased sensitivity and specificity as compared with creatine kinase–myoglobin (CK-MB) and total creatine kinase (CK). Troponin is more consistently elevated in acute MIs than CK-MB. Also, CK is found in many body tissues, and can, therefore, be elevated for various reasons. CK-MB is more specific for cardiac muscle than total CK, but it is also found in skeletal muscle, making it a less specific marker than troponin. Troponin also has enhanced prognostic value as compared to CK. B-type natriuretic peptide is a hormone used for evaluation of heart failure, not acute MI.

15. A: Dialysate is used with continuous venovenous hemodialysis (CVVHD) and continuous venovenous hemodiafiltration (CVVHDF) in order to remove solutes using the process of diffusion. CVVH removes solutes by creating a pressure gradient via convection without dialysate. Replacement fluid is used to aid in the flow of blood through the hemofilter. Ultrafiltrate is the fluid removed per hour.

16. B: Stress-induced (takotsubo) cardiomyopathy is characterized by transient systolic dysfunction of the apical segment of the left ventricle (LV), LV apical ballooning, electrocardiographic changes, mild elevation of troponin and cardiac enzymes, and absence of obstructive coronary artery disease. Symptoms may be similar to a myocardial infarction, but the fact that there is only very mild elevation in troponin and the patient's quick recovery should initiate the consideration of other options. The combination of characteristic findings described here and the preceding stressor indicate stress-induced cardiomyopathy. It is frequently triggered by an acute medical illness or an intense emotional or physical stress.

17. C: It is very important to obtain blood samples before antibiotic therapy to increase the likelihood of identifying the infecting organism. In patients who are acutely ill, three separate blood cultures should be obtained over a 1-hour period, and then empiric antibiotic therapy should be started. Once the organism is identified, the patient can be switched over to more specific antimicrobial agents. If the illness is subacute and the patient is not critically ill, three blood cultures should still be obtained before antibiotic therapy, but they can be collected over a longer period of time. In these subacute cases, it may be preferable to delay therapy for 1–3 days until the results of the blood cultures are back.

18. B: The patient requires extensive support and is unable to be weaned from the ventilator and venovenous extracorporeal membrane oxygenation. As a result, the patient will need a tracheostomy to prevent endotracheal tube-induced vocal cord damage and to increase oxygenation. This patient is in respiratory failure and does not need an LVAD, which is used in patients with end-stage heart failure. Plasmapheresis is a method of exchanging certain blood products to remove disease-causing antibodies; this procedure is usually used to treat autoimmune conditions and would not be beneficial for this patient. The patient is still in the early stages of illness and may recover without the need for a lung transplant.

19. C: Epoprostenol is a prostaglandin that treats pulmonary hypertension by dilating blood vessels in the lungs. Nausea and vomiting are possible side effects of epoprostenol escalation, and they can be a dose-limiting complication. The provider should be notified because the medication titration may need to be slowed or paused. Although bronchospasm may occur with inhaled epoprostenol, it is not a typical side effect on injected epoprostenol. Sudden hearing loss is not typically associated with epoprostenol, although sudden changes in vision can occur and should be reported. The patient is more at risk for hypotension than hypertension while the dose is being escalated.

20. A: The patient is demonstrating symptoms of an adrenal crisis, which include fatigue, weakness, nausea, flank pain, and hypotension. The patient is at a heightened risk for this condition due to a history of Addison's disease. This is an emergent situation that requires immediate administration of steroids via IV or intramuscularly to correct the endocrine imbalance. An abdominal computed tomography scan or nasogastric tube would be indicated if the provider were concerned about a bowel obstruction. The urine sample would be indicated if the provider were concerned about a urinary tract infection. However, because patients experiencing an adrenal crisis can rapidly deteriorate, the nurse would expect to the provider to address the adrenal crisis first.

21. D: Dilated cardiomyopathy can lead to heart failure as a result of ventricular dilation without cardiac muscle wall thickening. Verapamil should be questioned because it is a calcium channel blocker with negative inotropic effects, which can worsen heart failure. The patient has increased preload evidenced by a central venous pressure measurement of 24 and jugular venous distension. Furosemide is used to reduce preload. Amiodarone is an antiarrhythmic drug used to treat the patient's atrial fibrillation. Warfarin is an anticoagulant used to prevent thrombi (i.e., blood clots).

22. B: Clotting in the line would cause a high-venous-pressure alarm as a result of clots obstructing the blood flow within the circuit. Low blood pressure or hypovolemia would cause a low-arterial-pressure alarm. Air bubbles would cause an air-bubble-in-circuit alarm. Too much fluid removal could also cause a low-arterial-pressure alarm.

23. A: The patient is likely experiencing a retroperitoneal bleed. It is most important to replace volume loss until a blood transfusion can be given, if indicated. Replacing volume loss can also help raise the blood pressure. Norepinephrine can be indicated for hypotension, but less so in the context of hypotension secondary to hypovolemia. Collecting blood for a complete blood count and administering pain medication should follow the bolus because it is more important to first stabilize the patient by replacing volume.

24. C: Since the patient appears well and is breathing comfortably, her pulse oximetry should be rechecked (possibly with a different pulse oximeter) before further action is taken. The nurse should always consider the patient's physical state instead of just relying on test values. If the patient's oxygen saturation is actually low, then she can be started on oxygen, and her physician can be contacted about the change.

25. A: Unstable angina is one presentation of acute coronary syndrome. It is often reported as chest discomfort that is difficult to describe but may feel like tightness, squeezing, pressure, or aching in the chest. There may be radiation of the pain to the shoulder, arm, jaw, and neck as well as shortness of breath and sweating. Unstable angina may occur at rest without any instigation (e.g., while sleeping) and may last longer than 20 minutes. Answer B describes a typical presentation of chest pain due to pericarditis. Answer C describes a typical presentation of stable angina. Answer D describes a possible presentation of costochondritis.

26. D: The patient described in the question is experiencing a hypertensive emergency with associated hypertensive encephalopathy. In this situation, a patient's diastolic blood pressure should be rapidly lowered to around 100 mmHg with intravenous antihypertensive medication (with the maximum initial decrease 25% or less of the presenting value). This initial decrease in blood pressure should take place over 2–6 hours. Once the blood pressure is controlled, the patient should be switched to oral therapy, and the diastolic blood pressure should gradually be reduced to about 85 mmHg over the next 2–3 months. While the severity of the symptoms calls for rapid lowering of the blood pressure, if the blood pressure is lowered too much over a short period of time, other complications, such as renal failure, could occur.

27. B: The preferred reperfusion therapy for patients with an acute ST-segment elevation myocardial infarction is percutaneous coronary intervention (PCI). Fibrinolytic therapy is usually reserved for patients who cannot receive PCI in a timely fashion. If a patient has hemodynamic instability or cardiogenic shock, PCI is the treatment of choice, even if the patient has already received fibrinolytic therapy. Not all patients will need PCI after fibrinolytic therapy. If PCI is deemed necessary, it should not be performed within the first 2 hours after the administration of fibrinolytic therapy if possible. For stable patients who are subsequently found to have an occluded infarct-related artery, it is not recommended that PCI be performed if they do not show evidence of spontaneous or significant provocable ischemia.

28. A: Most cases of heparin-induced thrombocytopenia occur within 5–10 days of initiating heparin therapy. It is unusual to see onset after 2 weeks.

29. C: Carotid endarterectomy is a procedure that involves the removal of plaque from inside the carotid arteries in order to treat carotid stenosis. Postoperative hypertension can lead to stroke resulting from hyperperfusion. Hydralazine is the appropriate antihypertensive in the setting of bradycardia. The patient has a history of COPD, and an oxygen saturation of 93% is appropriate to prevent bradypnea. Labetalol is not appropriate in the setting of bradycardia. The patient's temperature is slightly elevated, but this is a common inflammatory response after surgery not requiring antipyretics.

30. C: Torsade de pointes is a distinctive form of polymorphic ventricular tachycardia in which there is a gradual change in the amplitude and twisting of the QRS complexes around the isoelectric line. It is associated with a congenital or acquired prolonged QT interval.

31. B: The American College of Cardiology/American Heart Association guidelines recommend that primary percutaneous coronary intervention (PCI) be implemented within 90 minutes of first medical contact in patients with ST-segment elevation myocardial infarctions who are otherwise eligible for the procedure. Studies have shown enhanced survival with PCI as compared to fibrinolysis.

32. C: Transcutaneous pacing is a method of depolarizing the heart to trigger a heartbeat and improve cardiac output via electrodes placed on the chest externally and is indicated in the context of a complete, or third-degree, heart block in which the atrium and ventricles are not communicating and the heart is not beating at a pace that provides sufficient perfusion to the body. Atropine may be used, but it acts at the atrioventricular (AV) node; as a result, it is usually not effective in treating third-degree heart block because, in this type of heart block, there is a lack of communication between the atrium and the ventricle. Amiodarone is an antiarrhythmic drug and will worsen bradycardia. Cardioversion is not used in third-degree heart block because conduction correction cannot take place due to the absence of communication between the sinoatrial (SA) and AV nodes.

33. D: The patient described in the question has inadequate perfusion along with signs and symptoms of volume overload. Cardiac output should be improved first, before excess volume is removed. Cardiac output can be increased by using intravenous vasodilators, inotropes, or both. In this case, a vasodilator may worsen hypotension, making the inotrope the appropriate intervention. After cardiac output is improved, diuretics can be used to address volume overload. Angiotensin-converting enzyme inhibitors will not address the patient's acute symptoms.

34. C: Patients undergoing the transfemoral TAVR approach should lie flat for 6 hours to maintain hemostasis at the access site and prevent bleeding. The patient will not need to take clopidogrel for life, but he will need to take aspirin for the remainder of his life to prevent clotting. Left arm restrictions are necessary when the subclavian approach is taken.

35. D: The range of normal arterial blood gas values varies slightly between laboratories, but the normal ranges are as follows: pH, 7.35–7.45; PCO_2, 35–45 mmHg; PaO_2, >80 mmHg (if new values are substantially different from old values then they may be considered abnormal even if more than 80 mmHg); and HCO_3, 21–27 mEq/L.

36. B: In the setting of an acute ischemic stroke, the current recommendation is to allow hypertension up to 220/120 mmHg in order to maximize perfusion to the brain, referred to as permissive hypertension. Should the patient's blood pressure exceed this limit, an IV antihypertensive agent (such as labetalol or nicardipine) is generally administered and titrated to a goal blood pressure. The blood pressure is maintained at a lower threshold if the patient is a candidate for thrombolytic therapy, such as tissue plasminogen activator, due to the risk of hemorrhage at higher blood pressures.

37. D: After receiving an arterial bypass, patients are at risk for complications such as compartment syndrome. The patient is demonstrating several of the classic symptoms of compartment syndrome (i.e., the five Ps: pain, pallor, pulselessness, paresthesia, paralysis), and the nurse should recognize these signs and notify the provider immediately. Although graft failure is a risk of peripheral artery bypass, this would typically develop over months or years after the procedure. Patients receiving an arterial bypass procedure are at risk for damage to their peripheral nerve, but this would result in alterations in pulses or skin color. Symptoms of a deep vein thrombosis would differ from those of compartment syndrome and include redness, warmth, and swelling at the site.

38. A: Grade I heart murmurs are very faint, but with practice, they can be heard when concentrating. Grade II murmurs are still faint but are more easily heard. Grade III murmurs are moderately loud and not associated with a thrill. Grade IV murmurs are loud and may be associated with a thrill. Grade V murmurs are very loud and associated with a thrill. Grade VI murmurs are very loud, can be heard even without a stethoscope on the chest, and are associated with a thrill.

39. A: Hypertension itself is not a risk factor associated with pneumothoraces. Men are more likely than women to develop pneumothoraces. Mechanical ventilation can cause an imbalance of air pressure in the chest, resulting in a pneumothorax. Smoking can damage lung tissue, and damaged lung tissue is more likely to collapse. Many underlying lung diseases or chest injuries may lead to pneumothoraces.

40. B: The patient is showing signs of a non-ST-elevation MI (NSTEMI), which should be treated but does not require emergent catheterization. The goal time for catheterization in the context of an NSTEMI is risk and symptom dependent but is typically recommended within 12–48 hours from the onset of symptoms, whereas the goal time for a patient suffering a STEMI would be 90 minutes.

41. D: Acute respiratory distress syndrome (ARDS) is a type of hypoxemic respiratory failure caused by acute, diffuse, inflammatory lung injury in both lungs. An important part of the care for patients with ARDS involves management of hypoxemia. This is done by using high fractions of inspired oxygen, decreasing oxygen consumption, improving oxygen delivery, and careful use of mechanical ventilatory support. In this case, sedating the patient will help to relieve anxiety and agitation and maximize rest, therefore, lowering oxygen consumption. Benzodiazepines do not act as analgesics.

42. B: If a patient with a pericardial effusion is hemodynamically stable and has no evidence of cardiac tamponade, immediate drainage of the effusion is not required. The underlying cause of the effusion should be determined and appropriate medical treatment instituted. If it is determined that the patient is stable, she can be treated as an outpatient. She should be educated about symptoms of increasing pericardial effusion, and outpatient follow-up should be scheduled.

43. A: Due to the cycling of blood outside body, the patient is at risk for hypothermia once the blood is returned to the body if the dialysis machine does not keep the blood adequately warm. The nurse should closely monitor the patient's temperature. Pulmonary edema and pruritus are not known complications of continuous renal replacement therapy. The patient is more at risk for hypotension than hypertension due to the removal of fluid from the body.

44. D: Diltiazem is a calcium channel blocking medication (aka a class IV antidysrhythmic). Its use results in smooth muscle relaxation and a subsequent reduction in force on the heart, which can lead to a lower heart rate in the setting of certain dysrhythmias, such as atrial fibrillation. Amiodarone is a potassium channel blocker, propranolol is a beta-adrenergic blocker, and lidocaine is a sodium channel blocker.

45. A: Cardiogenic shock is caused by cardiac pump failure, leading to decreased cardiac output and the inability to maintain perfusion to the vital organs. Decreased cardiac output can result in pulmonary congestion and pulmonary edema, resulting in crackles in the lungs. In hypovolemic and distributive shock there is more likely to be decreased jugular venous pressure (JVP), while in cardiogenic shock, increased JVP is often present.

46. D: The three major medical complications of acute myocardial infarction include rupture of the left ventricular free wall, rupture of the interventricular septum, and the development of mitral regurgitation (often due to papillary muscle rupture). If a new murmur develops, if there is evidence of hypoperfusion, or if severe decompensated heart failure occurs, suspicion of a mechanical complication is warranted. The diagnosis is often made with echocardiography. Each of these complications can lead to cardiogenic shock and death if not treated emergently.

47. C: Suction events cause the inner cannula of the LVAD to attach to the ventricular septum. It can occur when the ventricular pressure is too low as a result of hypovolemia, incorrect device positioning, or increased pump speed. Suction events can lead to arrhythmias. Infections occur as a result of the introduction of bacteria to the patient via lines and devices. Hypertension would be the result of hypervolemia. Pump thrombus occurs when anticoagulation has not been adequately achieved.

48. D: Transesophageal echocardiography (TEE) should be the initial test of choice in certain life-threatening situations or in cases where transthoracic echocardiography (TTE) is likely to be non-diagnostic. Examples where TEE should be the initial test include: suspected acute aortic pathology, suspected prosthetic valve dysfunction, suspected complications of endocarditis, and evaluation for thrombi in the left atrium. There are many more cases where TEE may be helpful, but often TTE is done first since it is a safer and less complicated test.

49. D: The patient is showing several signs of cardiac tamponade: quiet muffled heart sounds, jugular venous distension despite low blood pressure, pulsus paradoxus (a drop in blood pressure with inhalation), and a decreased pulse pressure (~25 mmHg with a normal pulse pressure of ~40 mmHg). Furthermore, with a known infection affecting the heart, the patient is at risk for developing fluid around the heart. Although a tension pneumothorax can cause similar symptoms, the nurse would expect to auscultate silent or diminished lung sounds in the affected lobes. Acute congestive heart failure can cause low blood pressure, decreased pulse pressure, and jugular vein distension; however, it would be unusual to see pulsus paradoxus, and the nurse would expect to auscultate fluid in the lungs. Mitral valve prolapse will also cause a murmur, but this condition is typically chronic and develops slowly and would not likely lead to the other acute changes experienced by this patient.

50. C: Subglottic suctioning will help reduce the risk of ventilator-acquired pneumonia associated with contaminated secretions reaching the lungs. Intubated patients are unable to use the incentive spirometer. Ventilator circuits should not be changed more frequently than every 48 hours in order to prevent infection. While turning the patient every 2 hours is an important component of caring for ventilated patients, the purpose of this intervention is to prevent pressure injuries rather than ventilator-acquired pneumonia.

51. A: Patients excluded from exercise electrocardiogram (ECG) include those who are unable to exercise sufficiently (to 85% of their predicted maximal heart rate) or those who have ECG abnormalities at rest that would interfere with test interpretation. The ECG abnormalities that exclude exercise ECG testing include the Wolff-Parkinson-White syndrome, a paced ventricular rhythm, complete left bundle branch block, more than 1 mm of ST depression at rest, ECG criteria for left ventricular hypertrophy, and patients taking digoxin. Patients who have a right bundle branch block are still candidates for diagnostic exercise ECG.

52. C: Patients should avoid submerging fully in water until their incision is healed (typically the first 4–12 weeks), but after that time, patients can return to swimming or taking a bath. Patients should avoid lifting the arm for at least the first 24 hours, and they should avoid picking up anything heavier than 10 pounds for the first 2 weeks to allow for proper healing. Although it may be sufficient for patients to call the clinic directly if they receive just a single shock with no complicating factors, patients should be told to call 911 immediately if they receive multiple shocks or if they receive a single shock and feel poorly, feel chest pain, or lose consciousness.

53. A: The patient should be rewarmed more slowly—at a rate of approximately 0.3 °C/hr. Bladder and esophageal temperatures are core measures and should be used with targeted temperature management. The targeted temperature for cooling is 32 °C as quickly as possible to reduce metabolic activity. Cisatracurium is a neuromuscular blocking drug used to prevent shivering (also to reduce metabolic activity) and ventilator dyssynchrony.

54. C: In pericarditis, there is J-point elevation and ST-segment elevation, which has a concave morphology that is usually diffusely seen in all leads. ST-segment elevation associated with acute myocardial infarction typically shows up in the leads corresponding to the area of infarction, rather than diffusely. The electrocardiogram in cardiac tamponade typically shows sinus tachycardia and low voltage. With left ventricular hypertrophy, ST–T-wave abnormalities are most often seen in anterolateral leads and typically consist of a horizontal or down sloping ST-segment and T-wave inversions.

55. D: Following a transradial catheterization, the patient is at risk of radial artery occlusion. The occlusion is not often visibly apparent or symptomatic due to collateral blood flow through the ulnar artery, but it can ultimately lead to hand ischemia. The nurse should assess for adequate blood flow through the radial artery by completing the reverse Barbeau test: The nurse occludes the ulnar artery of the affected hand while a pulse oximeter is placed on the thumb or forefinger of the same hand. The nurse observes the plethysmograph waveform of the pulse oximetry reading once the ulnar artery is occluded: If the waveform goes flat, it indicates reduced or absent blood flow through the radial artery; alternately, if the waveform continues as normal, it indicates adequate blood flow through the radial artery. The Barbeau test is completed in the same way but by manually occluding the radial artery to assess blood flow through the ulnar artery—this would be completed **prior to transradial catheterization** to ensure that the hand receives adequate blood supply through the ulnar artery. The palmar grasp and brachioradialis reflex tests would be completed as part of a neurological exam and would not be used following catheterization.

56. B: Torsade de pointes associated with hypokalemia is likely reversible once the electrolyte imbalances are corrected. Permanent pacing is considered definitely beneficial and effective in patients with symptomatic sinus bradycardia, second-degree atrioventricular Mobitz II block (especially if symptomatic), or significant carotid sinus hypersensitivity.

57. C: The patient is demonstrating signs of pulmonary edema—hypoxia, tachypnea, fine crackles, and pink frothy sputum—which is a potential complication of MI. The nurse should anticipate receiving an order for furosemide to address the excess fluid in the lungs. Ceftriaxone would be appropriate if the patient had pneumonia; however, due to a lack of a fever or other clinical indicators, pneumonia is not the most likely cause in this situation. A chest tube would be indicated if there were fluid or air collecting in the pleural space of the lung (such as in a hemothorax or pneumothorax); however, in pulmonary edema, there is an increase in extravascular fluid throughout the lungs, so a chest tube would not be helpful. Although some patients with pulmonary edema do require mechanical ventilation, this would not be indicated unless other, less invasive, interventions were ineffective or if the patient's condition became critically unstable.

58. C: The patient's telemetry monitor shows that he is experiencing torsades de pointes, a type of ventricular tachycardia typically caused by a prolonged QT. IV magnesium sulfate is the first-line drug used to reverse the underlying prolonged QT. Because the patient has a pulse, he would not be defibrillated. However, because he is hemodynamically compromised, the team should prepare to complete synchronized cardioversion. Amiodarone should not be given to a patient with torsades de pointes, which could further prolong the QT segment. Defibrillation would only be completed if the patient becomes pulseless.

59. B: In a patient with cocaine-associated acute myocardial ischemia or infarction, beta-blockers should not be used until the cocaine is eliminated from the body due to the risk of unopposed alpha-adrenergic stimulation. Unopposed alpha-adrenergic stimulation could lead to coronary artery vasoconstriction and systemic hypertension, causing worsening of the patient's condition. Aspirin, nitroglycerin, and oxygen remain safe and effective medications in cocaine-associated acute coronary syndrome cases.

60. C: Methemoglobinemia occurs when hemoglobin loses its iron molecule, forming methemoglobin, which is incapable of binding and carrying oxygen to the cells. Inhaled nitric oxide produces vasodilation of the pulmonary vasculature. It does not cause hypercapnia, oxygen toxicity, or volume overload

61. C: Pulmonary hypertension is a severe and progressive pulmonary disease that causes constriction of the pulmonary vasculature and increased resistance in the pulmonary vessels. Nitrous oxide is used to dilate the vessels and reduce the pressure within the pulmonary arteries. Furosemide is used in pulmonary hypertension to reduce volume overload when present. Pulmonary hypertension treatment does not target bicarbonate levels. Anticoagulants are used to prevent deep vein thrombosis and pulmonary embolism.

62. A: A 0.9% sodium chloride bolus should not be used in this patient because the ARDS has damaged the lung epithelium and caused pulmonary edema as evidenced by the chest x-ray. Fluids would worsen the pulmonary edema. Proning the patient helps recruit a greater surface area of lung tissue to improve oxygenation and ventilation-perfusion matching. Tube feeding the patient, even at minimal rates, helps prevent complications such as ileus and bacterial translocation. Maintaining plateau pressures helps prevent barotrauma.

63. C: The patient is demonstrating signs of acute pericarditis (i.e., chest pain that is relieved when sitting up, a pericardial friction rub, and ST segment changes generalized in all leads). The patient also has a significant risk factor for acute pericarditis after suffering an MI within the previous 72 hours. The first-line treatment for acute pericarditis is nonsteroidal anti-inflammatory drugs. The other options would be appropriate if the patient were having an MI.

64. B: In order to address the patient's hypoxia and increased oxygen requirements, the nurse would expect a gradual increase in both FiO_2 and PEEP. PEEP is increased to prevent alveolar collapse; however, if it is increased too drastically, it could put the patient at risk for barotrauma. If the FiO_2 is increased too drastically, it could lead to difficulties titrating it down later in the patient's treatment.

65. D: The acute change in blood pressure of the patient described in the question should be addressed immediately by establishing intravenous access with a large-bore intravenous catheter for the administration of fluids. As long as there is no evidence of pulmonary edema, a normal saline bolus should be given, and the patient should have a work-up for possible causes of the acute hypotension. The normal oxygen saturation is reassuring but should continue to be monitored. An arterial blood gas should be drawn, but establishing intravenous access is a priority. Nitroglycerin could worsen the patient's acute hypotension.

66. B: Angiotensin-converting enzyme (ACE) inhibitors not only help control blood pressure by causing vasodilation, but they also provide extra cardiac protection beyond that of other antihypertensive medications. The reduction in vascular tone leads to improved emptying of the left ventricle. The ACE inhibitors have also been shown to attenuate the remodeling process of the ventricles that is associated with congestive heart failure.

67. C: The patient described in the question most likely has a massive pulmonary embolus. Since the patient has persistent hypotension, thrombolytic therapy should be considered immediately with the aim of dissolving the embolism. Another immediate and potentially life-saving treatment option would be pulmonary arteriotomy with embolectomy. If the patient is hemodynamically stable and has no contraindications, therapy with heparin or low-molecular-weight heparin should be started for fast anticoagulation. Oral warfarin should be started on day 1, but this medication will generally take several days to achieve appropriate anticoagulation. A ventilation/perfusion scan or computed tomography pulmonary angiogram can be performed after the patient is stable to confirm the diagnosis of pulmonary embolism.

68. A: In an asymptomatic patient with a descending thoracic aortic aneurysm with a diameter of less than 6 cm, medical management is generally recommended, though some evidence is showing that the individual's height should also be taken into account when considering surgery. Medical management includes aggressive blood pressure control with beta-blockers as part of the regimen, surveillance for signs and symptoms, and serial imaging to evaluate growth and structure. Surgery is indicated if the patient is symptomatic, if the descending aortic aneurysm is 6 cm or greater, if the aneurysm has an accelerated growth rate, or if there is evidence of dissection.

69. B: The patient's pulmonary artery catheter (aka Swan-Ganz catheter) readings reveal a diagnosis of congestive heart failure. A fluid bolus will worsen the cardiac pressures by increasing preload and the pulmonary arterial wedge pressure. Dobutamine is given to increase the contractility of the heart, furosemide to reduce preload, and norepinephrine to increase the blood pressure.

70. A: Atrial fibrillation has been shown to occur in up to 60% of binge drinkers, even if they did not have underlying alcoholic cardiomyopathy. Regular heavy alcohol consumption is also associated with an increase in the occurrence of atrial fibrillation.

71. C: There are no physical examination findings that can definitively diagnose a deep venous thrombosis (DVT), but certain findings may help guide further action. Findings that may be associated with a DVT include a palpable cord, unilateral calf or thigh pain, unilateral edema, warmth, tenderness, erythema, and superficial venous dilation. Skin breakdown is not a typical sign of DVT.

72. D: Ventricular fibrillation is caused by rapid discharges from many irritable ventricular automaticity foci. This produces an irregular, rapid twitching of the ventricles, resulting in an erratic electrocardiographic (ECG) tracing with no distinguishable waves. Atrial flutter is characterized by a series of identical, rapid "flutter" waves (often described as a "saw tooth" pattern) with distinguishable, but possibly irregular QRS complexes. Atrial fibrillation often appears as a wavy baseline without distinguishable P waves and an irregular QRS response. Ventricular flutter appears as a rapid series of smooth sine waves of similar amplitude on ECG.

73. C: In some patients with persistent atrial fibrillation, cardioversion to sinus rhythm is a treatment option. It is recommended that a patient be anticoagulated for 3–4 weeks before and after cardioversion to reduce the risk of thromboembolism. If it is decided that cardioversion should be done sooner, before therapeutic anticoagulation is achieved, then a transesophageal echocardiogram should be done before cardioversion to exclude the presence of an existing intracardiac thrombus.

74. B: Differences in treating patients with acute myocardial infarction complicated by cardiogenic shock as compared to treating patients without shock include holding clopidogrel until after angiography, using lidocaine in low doses, and avoiding drugs with negative inotropic properties, such as beta-blockers and calcium channel blockers, while the patient is in shock. The patient can still be treated with aspirin.

75. B: Risk factors for developing torsade de pointes include certain electrolyte disturbances, especially hypomagnesemia and hypokalemia. Less often hypocalcemia is found to be a cause. A first-line therapy for the treatment of torsade de pointes is intravenous magnesium sulfate. It is effective for both the treatment and prevention of the long QT-related arrhythmia. These treatments have been shown to be beneficial even in patients with normal baseline serum magnesium concentrations.

76. B: Because the patient's current vital signs are all within the normal range and the left ventricular ejection fraction is greater than 25%, the patient is ready to receive less support from the IABP. Standard care typically includes reducing IABP support from 1:1 to 1:2 to 1:3. The IABP would not be removed until the patient continues to demonstrate stable vital signs while receiving less support. It is not possible to increase IABP support beyond 1:1.

77. B: Continuous positive airway pressure (CPAP) is contraindicated in patients who are suspected of having a pneumothorax, because the CPAP would likely cause an increased buildup of air (and therefore tension) in the chest cavity, which may result in further deterioration of the patient's condition. CPAP has been shown to be helpful as noninvasive positive pressure ventilation in other causes of acute respiratory failure, such as cardiogenic pulmonary edema, pneumonia, and chronic obstructive pulmonary disease.

78. B: Stroke is the most serious acute complication associated with coronary artery stenting in patients with carotid stenosis. Stroke may result from thromboembolism, hypoperfusion, intracerebral hemorrhage, or cerebral hyperperfusion. Stent fractures, myocardial infarctions, and renal dysfunction are other complications of coronary artery stenting, but stroke is considered the most serious.

79. C: Morphine eases the work of breathing and the sensation of shortness of breath by reducing the respiration rate and prolonging expiration, which decreases air hunger and the sensation of breathlessness. It is commonly used to treat symptoms of shortness of breath at the end of life. Morphine will not decrease the patient's congestion. Morphine can be used to treat pain, but it does not prevent pain and should not be taken prophylactically due to its possible side effects.

80. B: Cor pulmonale refers to the altered structure and function of the right ventricle of the heart. This dysfunction can result from any cause of pulmonary hypertension. Typically, cor pulmonale is slowly progressive, but in some cases, it can be acute. Symptoms include dyspnea on exertion, fatigue, exertional angina, and syncope.

81. C: This patient is experiencing respiratory acidosis due to insufficient ventilation. The set rate would likely be increased to allow the patient to blow off the excessive CO_2. The PaO_2 is within normal limits; therefore, increasing the PEEP or FiO_2 is not indicated. Reducing the set rate will worsen the retainment of CO_2 and therefore worsen the patient's acidosis.

82. A: The patient described in the question has experienced occlusion of his mesenteric artery with resultant intestinal ischemia. This complication is caused by trauma to a blood vessel or by dislodging an atherosclerotic plaque in the vessel. Systemic embolization caused by cardiac catheterization can cause cutaneous, renal, retinal, cerebral, or gastrointestinal emboli, which may or may not be clinically significant. Although renal dysfunction may be caused by a renal embolus, the bloody diarrhea and sudden onset of diffuse abdominal pain in this case make it more likely that mesenteric ischemia is the cause. Cholecystitis and gastric ulceration are not complications related to cardiac catheterization.

83. C: An international normalized ratio between 2 and 3 is recommended for most patients with atrial fibrillation to prevent embolization of atrial thrombi. If the patient has other risk factors, his target range may need to be adjusted.

84. C: When a patient has a bradyarrhythmia with a pulse, it is important to determine whether the bradyarrhythmia is causing hypotension, acutely altered mental status, signs of shock, ischemic chest discomfort, or acute heart failure. If none of these signs or symptoms is present, the patient can be monitored and observed. If one or more of these sign or symptoms is present, such as in this scenario, a 1 mg bolus of intravenous atropine should be given every 3–5 minutes (to a maximum of 3 mg). If atropine is ineffective, transcutaneous pacing, a dopamine infusion, or an epinephrine infusion should be considered.

85. A: One of the main purposes of targeted temperature management (TTM) after a resuscitated cardiac arrest is to improve neurological outcomes. Neurologic injury is the most common cause of death in patients who experience a cardiac arrest while not in the hospital.

86. D: A first-degree atrioventricular (AV) block is defined as a prolonged PR interval (> 0.20 seconds), resulting in slowed AV conduction. A second-degree AV Mobitz I block is the result of an intermittent block of the impulse within the AV node. The electrocardiogram shows progressive lengthening of the PR interval so that a normally occurring P wave is not followed by a QRS complex, and then the cycle begins again. A second-degree AV Mobitz II block is characterized by unpredictable failure of AV conduction. There is no change in the PR interval before or after the non-conducted P wave. A third-degree AV block occurs when there is complete failure of the AV node to conduct any impulses from the atria to the ventricles. This results in a disconnect between the atrial rhythm and the ventricular rhythm.

87. B: All patients who receive an LVAD are at a high risk for thrombotic events and are on lifelong anticoagulation therapy. Although anticoagulants always pose a risk of internal bleeding, the risk of bleeding from the driveline site is small once the surgical incision has healed, and this is not a reason to avoid blood thinners. The patient or a caregiver will be responsible for daily self-tests and regular dressing changes at home. The patient will also require proper fluid volume intake to prevent any complications of hypovolemia such as suction events and dysrhythmias.

88. D: Characteristic symptoms of cardiac tamponade include sinus tachycardia, hypotension, elevated jugular venous pressure (JVP), and pulsus paradoxus. Beat-to-beat alterations in the QRS complex seen on electrocardiogram (ECG), otherwise known as electrical alternans, are a relatively specific finding for cardiac tamponade. Hypotension and elevated JVP can be seen in cases of acute myocardial infarction (MI) and large pulmonary emboli; however, these disorders are not associated with pulsus paradoxus. In addition, acute MI is associated with characteristic ECG changes of infarction. Although aortic dissection may lead to the development of cardiac tamponade, aortic dissection in the absence of cardiac tamponade should not cause an increase in JVP.

89. A: the P-level should be reduced to P-2 during CPR to prevent damage to the heart structures. Defibrillation can be performed on a patient with an Impella device. CPR should be initiated based on perfusion and flow because the patient with an Impella device may still have flow in the presence of a flat arterial waveform. The Impella device does not need to be turned off during CPR.

90. D: Avoiding the ingestion of solids and liquids at the same time prevents the patient from swallowing food before it is chewed adequately. Avoid cold or hot foods and liquids because stroke patients may have extra sensitivity to hot and cold temperatures. Sticky foods are harder for the patient to manage and may cause pocketing and subsequent aspiration. Straws may cause the patient to aspirate because they can place liquids in the back of the throat, which causes difficulty with swallowing.

How to Overcome Test Anxiety

Just the thought of taking a test is enough to make most people a little nervous. A test is an important event that can have a long-term impact on your future, so it's important to take it seriously and it's natural to feel anxious about performing well. But just because anxiety is normal, that doesn't mean that it's helpful in test taking, or that you should simply accept it as part of your life. Anxiety can have a variety of effects. These effects can be mild, like making you feel slightly nervous, or severe, like blocking your ability to focus or remember even a simple detail.

If you experience test anxiety—whether severe or mild—it's important to know how to beat it. To discover this, first you need to understand what causes test anxiety.

Causes of Test Anxiety

While we often think of anxiety as an uncontrollable emotional state, it can actually be caused by simple, practical things. One of the most common causes of test anxiety is that a person does not feel adequately prepared for their test. This feeling can be the result of many different issues such as poor study habits or lack of organization, but the most common culprit is time management. Starting to study too late, failing to organize your study time to cover all of the material, or being distracted while you study will mean that you're not well prepared for the test. This may lead to cramming the night before, which will cause you to be physically and mentally exhausted for the test. Poor time management also contributes to feelings of stress, fear, and hopelessness as you realize you are not well prepared but don't know what to do about it.

Other times, test anxiety is not related to your preparation for the test but comes from unresolved fear. This may be a past failure on a test, or poor performance on tests in general. It may come from comparing yourself to others who seem to be performing better or from the stress of living up to expectations. Anxiety may be driven by fears of the future—how failure on this test would affect your educational and career goals. These fears are often completely irrational, but they can still negatively impact your test performance.

Elements of Test Anxiety

As mentioned earlier, test anxiety is considered to be an emotional state, but it has physical and mental components as well. Sometimes you may not even realize that you are suffering from test anxiety until you notice the physical symptoms. These can include trembling hands, rapid heartbeat, sweating, nausea, and tense muscles. Extreme anxiety may lead to fainting or vomiting. Obviously, any of these symptoms can have a negative impact on testing. It is important to recognize them as soon as they begin to occur so that you can address the problem before it damages your performance.

The mental components of test anxiety include trouble focusing and inability to remember learned information. During a test, your mind is on high alert, which can help you recall information and stay focused for an extended period of time. However, anxiety interferes with your mind's natural processes, causing you to blank out, even on the questions you know well. The strain of testing during anxiety makes it difficult to stay focused, especially on a test that may take several hours. Extreme anxiety can take a huge mental toll, making it difficult not only to recall test information but even to understand the test questions or pull your thoughts together.

Effects of Test Anxiety

Test anxiety is like a disease—if left untreated, it will get progressively worse. Anxiety leads to poor performance, and this reinforces the feelings of fear and failure, which in turn lead to poor performances on subsequent tests. It can grow from a mild nervousness to a crippling condition. If allowed to progress, test anxiety can have a big impact on your schooling, and consequently on your future.

Test anxiety can spread to other parts of your life. Anxiety on tests can become anxiety in any stressful situation, and blanking on a test can turn into panicking in a job situation. But fortunately, you don't have to let anxiety rule your testing and determine your grades. There are a number of relatively simple steps you can take to move past anxiety and function normally on a test and in the rest of life.

Physical Steps for Beating Test Anxiety

While test anxiety is a serious problem, the good news is that it can be overcome. It doesn't have to control your ability to think and remember information. While it may take time, you can begin taking steps today to beat anxiety.

Just as your first hint that you may be struggling with anxiety comes from the physical symptoms, the first step to treating it is also physical. Rest is crucial for having a clear, strong mind. If you are tired, it is much easier to give in to anxiety. But if you establish good sleep habits, your body and mind will be ready to perform optimally, without the strain of exhaustion. Additionally, sleeping well helps you to retain information better, so you're more likely to recall the answers when you see the test questions.

Getting good sleep means more than going to bed on time. It's important to allow your brain time to relax. Take study breaks from time to time so it doesn't get overworked, and don't study right before bed. Take time to rest your mind before trying to rest your body, or you may find it difficult to fall asleep.

Along with sleep, other aspects of physical health are important in preparing for a test. Good nutrition is vital for good brain function. Sugary foods and drinks may give a burst of energy but this burst is followed by a crash, both physically and emotionally. Instead, fuel your body with protein and vitamin-rich foods.

Also, drink plenty of water. Dehydration can lead to headaches and exhaustion, especially if your brain is already under stress from the rigors of the test. Particularly if your test is a long one, drink water during the breaks. And if possible, take an energy-boosting snack to eat between sections.

Along with sleep and diet, a third important part of physical health is exercise. Maintaining a steady workout schedule is helpful, but even taking 5-minute study breaks to walk can help get your blood pumping faster and clear your head. Exercise also releases endorphins, which contribute to a positive feeling and can help combat test anxiety.

When you nurture your physical health, you are also contributing to your mental health. If your body is healthy, your mind is much more likely to be healthy as well. So take time to rest, nourish your body with healthy food and water, and get moving as much as possible. Taking these physical steps will make you stronger and more able to take the mental steps necessary to overcome test anxiety.

Mental Steps for Beating Test Anxiety

Working on the mental side of test anxiety can be more challenging, but as with the physical side, there are clear steps you can take to overcome it. As mentioned earlier, test anxiety often stems from lack of preparation, so the obvious solution is to prepare for the test. Effective studying may be the most important weapon you have for beating test anxiety, but you can and should employ several other mental tools to combat fear.

First, boost your confidence by reminding yourself of past success—tests or projects that you aced. If you're putting as much effort into preparing for this test as you did for those, there's no reason you should expect to fail here. Work hard to prepare; then trust your preparation.

Second, surround yourself with encouraging people. It can be helpful to find a study group, but be sure that the people you're around will encourage a positive attitude. If you spend time with others who are anxious or cynical, this will only contribute to your own anxiety. Look for others who are motivated to study hard from a desire to succeed, not from a fear of failure.

Third, reward yourself. A test is physically and mentally tiring, even without anxiety, and it can be helpful to have something to look forward to. Plan an activity following the test, regardless of the outcome, such as going to a movie or getting ice cream.

When you are taking the test, if you find yourself beginning to feel anxious, remind yourself that you know the material. Visualize successfully completing the test. Then take a few deep, relaxing breaths and return to it. Work through the questions carefully but with confidence, knowing that you are capable of succeeding.

Developing a healthy mental approach to test taking will also aid in other areas of life. Test anxiety affects more than just the actual test—it can be damaging to your mental health and even contribute to depression. It's important to beat test anxiety before it becomes a problem for more than testing.

Study Strategy

Being prepared for the test is necessary to combat anxiety, but what does being prepared look like? You may study for hours on end and still not feel prepared. What you need is a strategy for test prep. The next few pages outline our recommended steps to help you plan out and conquer the challenge of preparation.

STEP 1: SCOPE OUT THE TEST

Learn everything you can about the format (multiple choice, essay, etc.) and what will be on the test. Gather any study materials, course outlines, or sample exams that may be available. Not only will this help you to prepare, but knowing what to expect can help to alleviate test anxiety.

STEP 2: MAP OUT THE MATERIAL

Look through the textbook or study guide and make note of how many chapters or sections it has. Then divide these over the time you have. For example, if a book has 15 chapters and you have five days to study, you need to cover three chapters each day. Even better, if you have the time, leave an extra day at the end for overall review after you have gone through the material in depth.

If time is limited, you may need to prioritize the material. Look through it and make note of which sections you think you already have a good grasp on, and which need review. While you are studying, skim quickly through the familiar sections and take more time on the challenging parts.

Write out your plan so you don't get lost as you go. Having a written plan also helps you feel more in control of the study, so anxiety is less likely to arise from feeling overwhelmed at the amount to cover.

STEP 3: GATHER YOUR TOOLS

Decide what study method works best for you. Do you prefer to highlight in the book as you study and then go back over the highlighted portions? Or do you type out notes of the important information? Or is it helpful to make flashcards that you can carry with you? Assemble the pens, index cards, highlighters, post-it notes, and any other materials you may need so you won't be distracted by getting up to find things while you study.

If you're having a hard time retaining the information or organizing your notes, experiment with different methods. For example, try color-coding by subject with colored pens, highlighters, or post-it notes. If you learn better by hearing, try recording yourself reading your notes so you can listen while in the car, working out, or simply sitting at your desk. Ask a friend to quiz you from your flashcards, or try teaching someone the material to solidify it in your mind.

STEP 4: CREATE YOUR ENVIRONMENT

It's important to avoid distractions while you study. This includes both the obvious distractions like visitors and the subtle distractions like an uncomfortable chair (or a too-comfortable couch that makes you want to fall asleep). Set up the best study environment possible: good lighting and a comfortable work area. If background music helps you focus, you may want to turn it on, but otherwise keep the room quiet. If you are using a computer to take notes, be sure you don't have any other windows open, especially applications like social media, games, or anything else that could distract you. Silence your phone and turn off notifications. Be sure to keep water close by so you stay hydrated while you study (but avoid unhealthy drinks and snacks).

Also, take into account the best time of day to study. Are you freshest first thing in the morning? Try to set aside some time then to work through the material. Is your mind clearer in the afternoon or evening? Schedule your study session then. Another method is to study at the same time of day that you will take the test, so that your brain gets used to working on the material at that time and will be ready to focus at test time.

STEP 5: STUDY!

Once you have done all the study preparation, it's time to settle into the actual studying. Sit down, take a few moments to settle your mind so you can focus, and begin to follow your study plan. Don't give in to distractions or let yourself procrastinate. This is your time to prepare so you'll be ready to fearlessly approach the test. Make the most of the time and stay focused.

Of course, you don't want to burn out. If you study too long you may find that you're not retaining the information very well. Take regular study breaks. For example, taking five minutes out of every hour to walk briskly, breathing deeply and swinging your arms, can help your mind stay fresh.

As you get to the end of each chapter or section, it's a good idea to do a quick review. Remind yourself of what you learned and work on any difficult parts. When you feel that you've mastered the material, move on to the next part. At the end of your study session, briefly skim through your notes again.

But while review is helpful, cramming last minute is NOT. If at all possible, work ahead so that you won't need to fit all your study into the last day. Cramming overloads your brain with more information than it can process and retain, and your tired mind may struggle to recall even previously learned information when it is overwhelmed with last-minute study. Also, the urgent nature of cramming and the stress placed on your brain contribute to anxiety. You'll be more likely to go to the test feeling unprepared and having trouble thinking clearly.

So don't cram, and don't stay up late before the test, even just to review your notes at a leisurely pace. Your brain needs rest more than it needs to go over the information again. In fact, plan to finish your studies by noon or early afternoon the day before the test. Give your brain the rest of the day to relax or focus on other things, and get a good night's sleep. Then you will be fresh for the test and better able to recall what you've studied.

STEP 6: TAKE A PRACTICE TEST

Many courses offer sample tests, either online or in the study materials. This is an excellent resource to check whether you have mastered the material, as well as to prepare for the test format and environment.

Check the test format ahead of time: the number of questions, the type (multiple choice, free response, etc.), and the time limit. Then create a plan for working through them. For example, if you have 30 minutes to take a 60-question test, your limit is 30 seconds per question. Spend less time on the questions you know well so that you can take more time on the difficult ones.

If you have time to take several practice tests, take the first one open book, with no time limit. Work through the questions at your own pace and make sure you fully understand them. Gradually work up to taking a test under test conditions: sit at a desk with all study materials put away and set a timer. Pace yourself to make sure you finish the test with time to spare and go back to check your answers if you have time.

After each test, check your answers. On the questions you missed, be sure you understand why you missed them. Did you misread the question (tests can use tricky wording)? Did you forget the information? Or was it something you hadn't learned? Go back and study any shaky areas that the practice tests reveal.

Taking these tests not only helps with your grade, but also aids in combating test anxiety. If you're already used to the test conditions, you're less likely to worry about it, and working through tests until you're scoring well gives you a confidence boost. Go through the practice tests until you feel comfortable, and then you can go into the test knowing that you're ready for it.

Test Tips

On test day, you should be confident, knowing that you've prepared well and are ready to answer the questions. But aside from preparation, there are several test day strategies you can employ to maximize your performance.

First, as stated before, get a good night's sleep the night before the test (and for several nights before that, if possible). Go into the test with a fresh, alert mind rather than staying up late to study.

Try not to change too much about your normal routine on the day of the test. It's important to eat a nutritious breakfast, but if you normally don't eat breakfast at all, consider eating just a protein bar. If you're a coffee drinker, go ahead and have your normal coffee. Just make sure you time it so that the caffeine doesn't wear off right in the middle of your test. Avoid sugary beverages, and drink enough water to stay hydrated but not so much that you need a restroom break 10 minutes into the test. If your test isn't first thing in the morning, consider going for a walk or doing a light workout before the test to get your blood flowing.

Allow yourself enough time to get ready, and leave for the test with plenty of time to spare so you won't have the anxiety of scrambling to arrive in time. Another reason to be early is to select a good seat. It's helpful to sit away from doors and windows, which can be distracting. Find a good seat, get out your supplies, and settle your mind before the test begins.

When the test begins, start by going over the instructions carefully, even if you already know what to expect. Make sure you avoid any careless mistakes by following the directions.

Then begin working through the questions, pacing yourself as you've practiced. If you're not sure on an answer, don't spend too much time on it, and don't let it shake your confidence. Either skip it and come back later, or eliminate as many wrong answers as possible and guess among the remaining ones. Don't dwell on these questions as you continue—put them out of your mind and focus on what lies ahead.

Be sure to read all of the answer choices, even if you're sure the first one is the right answer. Sometimes you'll find a better one if you keep reading. But don't second-guess yourself if you do immediately know the answer. Your gut instinct is usually right. Don't let test anxiety rob you of the information you know.

If you have time at the end of the test (and if the test format allows), go back and review your answers. Be cautious about changing any, since your first instinct tends to be correct, but make sure you didn't misread any of the questions or accidentally mark the wrong answer choice. Look over any you skipped and make an educated guess.

At the end, leave the test feeling confident. You've done your best, so don't waste time worrying about your performance or wishing you could change anything. Instead, celebrate the successful completion of this test. And finally, use this test to learn how to deal with anxiety even better next time.

> **Review Video: Test Anxiety**
> Visit mometrix.com/academy and enter code: 100340

Important Qualification

Not all anxiety is created equal. If your test anxiety is causing major issues in your life beyond the classroom or testing center, or if you are experiencing troubling physical symptoms related to your anxiety, it may be a sign of a serious physiological or psychological condition. If this sounds like your situation, we strongly encourage you to seek professional help.

Online Resources

Due to our efforts to try to keep this book to a manageable length, we've created a link that will give you access to all of your online resources:

mometrix.com/resources719/cmc-22549

It's Your Moment, Let's Celebrate It!

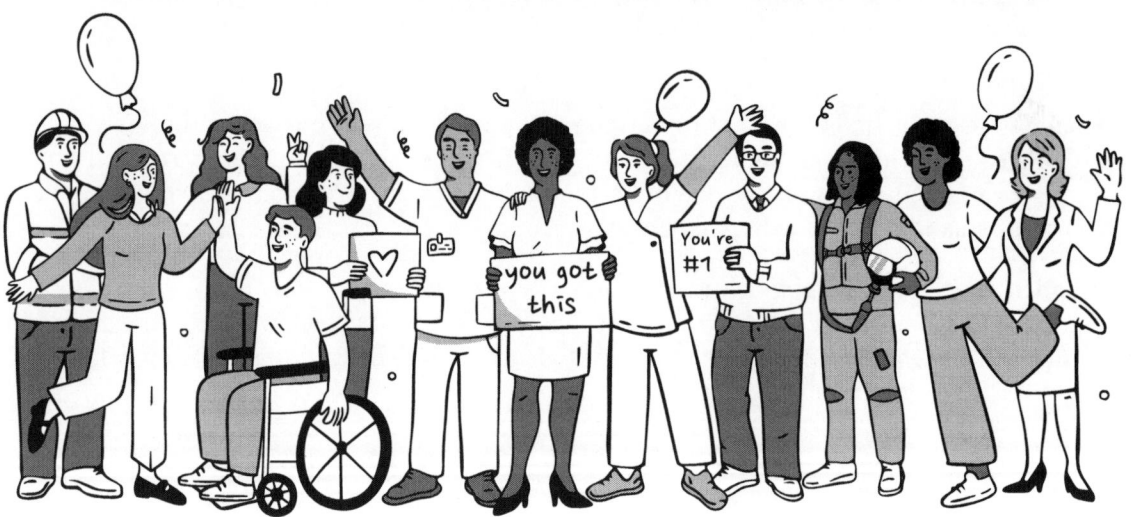

Share your story @mometrixtestpreparation